Positron-Emission Tomography in Schizophrenia Research

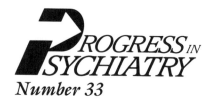

_PROGRESS__IN_
PSYCHIATRY
Number 33

David Spiegel, M.D.
Series Editor

Positron-Emission Tomography in Schizophrenia Research

Edited by
Nora D. Volkow, M.D.
Alfred P. Wolf, Ph.D.

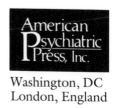

American Psychiatric Press, Inc.

Washington, DC
London, England

Note: The authors have worked to ensure that all information in this book concerning drug dosages, schedules, and routes of administration is accurate as of the time of publication and consistent with standards set by the U.S. Food and Drug Administration and the general medical community. As medical research and practice advance, however, therapeutic standards may change. For this reason and because human and mechanical errors sometimes occur, we recommend that readers follow the advice of a physician who is directly involved in their care or the care of a member of their family.

Copyright © 1991 American Psychiatric Press, Inc.
ALL RIGHTS RESERVED
Manufactured in the United States of America on acid-free paper.
First Printing 94 93 92 91 4 3 2 1

American Psychiatric Press, Inc.
1400 K Street, N.W., Washington, DC 20005

Library of Congress Cataloging-in-Publication Data

Positron-emission tomography in schizophrenia research/ edited by Nora D. Volkow, Alfred P. Wolf.
    p. cm.—(Progress in psychiatry ; no. 33)
   Includes bibliographical references.
   ISBN 0-88048-195-1 (alk. paper)
   1. Schizophrenia—Research. 2. Tomography, Emission.
3. Brain—Tomography. I. Volkow, Nora D., 1956-   . II. Wolf, Alfred P. III. Series.
   [DNLM: 1. Schizophrenia. 2. Tomography, Emission-Computed. WM 203 U84]
RC514.U84 1991
616.89′82072—dc20
DNLM/DLC
for Library of Congress   90-14487
                                            CIP

British Library Cataloguing in Publication Data

A CIP record is available from the British Library.

Contents

Contributors

Bernard Bendriem, Ph.D.
Chemistry Department, Brookhaven National Laboratory, Upton, New York

Jonathan D. Brodie, M.D., Ph.D.
Department of Psychiatry, New York University, New York, New York

Monte S. Buchsbaum, M.D.
Department of Psychiatry, Brain Imaging Center, University of California, Irvine

Robert Cancro, M.D.
Department of Psychiatry, New York University, New York, New York

Raquel E. Gur, M.D., Ph.D.
Brain Behavior Laboratory and the Neuropsychiatry Program, Departments of Psychiatry and Neurology, University of Pennsylvania, Philadelphia, Pennsylvania

Ruben C. Gur, Ph.D.
Brain Behavior Laboratory and the Neuropsychiatry Program, Departments of Psychiatry and Neurology, University of Pennsylvania, Philadelphia, Pennsylvania

David J. Schlyer, Ph.D.
Department of Chemistry, Brookhaven National Laboratory, Upton, New York

Nora D. Volkow, M.D.
Medical Department, Brookhaven National Laboratory, Upton, New York

Alfred P. Wolf, Ph.D.
Chemistry Department, Brookhaven National Laboratory, Upton, New York

Dean F. Wong, M.D.
Department of Radiology, Division of Nuclear Medicine, The Johns Hopkins Medical Institutions, Baltimore, Maryland

L. Trevor Young, M.D.
Department of Radiology, Division of Nuclear Medicine, The Johns Hopkins Medical Institutions, Baltimore, Maryland

Introduction to the Progress in Psychiatry Series

The Progress in Psychiatry Series is designed to capture in print the excitement that comes from assembling a diverse group of experts from various locations to examine in detail the newest information about a developing aspect of psychiatry. This series emerged as a collaboration between the American Psychiatric Association's (APA) Scientific Program Committee and the American Psychiatric Press, Inc. Great interest is generated by a number of the symposia presented each year at the APA annual meeting, and we realized that much of the information presented there, carefully assembled by people who are deeply immersed in a given area, would unfortunately not appear together in print. The symposia sessions at the annual meetings provide an unusual opportunity for experts who otherwise might not meet on the same platform to share their diverse viewpoints for a period of 3 hours. Some new themes are repeatedly reinforced and gain credence, while in other instances disagreements emerge, enabling the audience and now the reader to reach informed decisions about new directions in the field. The Progress in Psychiatry Series allows us to publish and capture some of the best of the symposia and thus provide an in-depth treatment of specific areas that might not otherwise be presented in broader review formats.

Psychiatry is by nature an interface discipline, combining the study of mind and brain, of individual and social environments, of the humane and the scientific. Therefore, progress in the field is rarely linear—it often comes from unexpected sources. Further, new developments emerge from an array of viewpoints that do not necessarily provide immediate agreement but rather expert examination of the issues. We intend to present innovative ideas and data that will enable you, the reader, to participate in this process.

We believe the Progress in Psychiatry Series will provide you with an opportunity to review timely new information in specific fields of interest as they are developing. We hope you find that the excitement of the presentations is captured in the written word and that this book proves to be informative and enjoyable reading.

David Spiegel, M.D.
Series Editor
Progress in Psychiatry Series

Progress in Psychiatry Series Titles

Current Concepts of Somatization: Research and Clinical Perspectives (#31)
Edited by Laurence J. Kirmayer, M.D., F.R.C.P.(C), and James M. Robbins, Ph.D.

Mental Retardation: Developing Pharmacotherapies (#32)
Edited by John J. Ratey, M.D.

Positron-Emission Tomography in Schizophrenia Research (#33)
Edited by Nora D. Volkow, M.D., and Alfred P. Wolf, Ph.D.

Brain Imaging in Affective Disorders (#34)
Edited by Peter Hauser, M.D.

Psychoimmunology Update (#35)
Edited by Jack M. Gorman, M.D., and Robert M. Kertzner, M.D.

Preface

The notion that schizophrenia is a result of organic brain pathology has motivated the search for abnormalities in the brains of schizophrenic patients. Although the etiopathogenesis of schizophrenic disorders is far from being elucidated, numerous abnormalities have already been described in these patients. Neuropathological studies have shown neuronal loss, vascular defects, gliosis, and demyelination in the brain of schizophrenic patients. The cortical areas more frequently reported as abnormal in the brains of schizophrenic patients are the frontal and the temporal cortices. Radiological studies using computed tomography scans and magnetic resonance imaging, although not always consistent, tend to report evidence of cortical atrophy and ventricular enlargement. In parallel to these morphological studies have been neurochemical studies attempting to uncover defects in neurotransmitters, receptors, and/or enzymes in the brains of schizophrenic patients. Because of the therapeutic efficacy of neuroleptics in schizophrenic disorders, work with neurotransmitters in schizophrenic patients has focused on the dopamine system. However, abnormalities in other neurotransmitter systems have also been proposed, with studies reporting decreases, increases, or no changes in norepinephrine, serotonin, gamma-aminobutyric acid, and opiates, among others. The great frequency with which discrepant results are reported in research in schizophrenia could reflect several factors: 1) the heterogeneous nature of the disease, 2) differences in experimental methodology, and 3) influence of developmental and environmental factors. However, these discrepancies can also represent a lack of an adequate technology to measure brain function and neurochemistry. Neurochemical measurements have typically been obtained indirectly by blood and/or urine analysis, or by performing the measurements on postmortem brains of schizophrenic patients.

Positron-emission tomography (PET) was first introduced into extensive clinical research in the late 1960s and early 1970s by pioneering groups at the Massachusetts General Hospital and Washington University, St. Louis. Dr. Bendriem, in Chapter 1, gives a brief overview of PET technology and how it is applied.

The first PET studies performed in schizophrenic patients were aimed at assessing functional brain abnormalities using ^{18}F-labeled fluorodeoxyglucose ($[^{18}$F]FDG). This approach followed very quickly after the first synthesis of [^{18}F]FDG reported by the Brookhaven National Laboratory (BNL) group in 1976. This work was the result of a collaborative effort among the University of Pennsylvania, BNL, and the National Institutes of Health (NIH). Its applicability in providing a quantitative measure of local cerebral glucose metabolism was based on the model developed by Dr. L. Sokoloff of NIH. The rate of glucose metabolism provides a measure of brain function, since in the normal brain the energy requirement for functional activation is mainly derived from glucose. The initial study applied to schizophrenia was reported in 1979 by Dr. Tibor Farkas working at BNL and New York University. In 1982, Dr. Buchsbaum, then at NIH, also demonstrated decreased glucose metabolism in the frontal cortex of schizophrenic patients. Since then, several centers have further investigated the significance and frequency of this abnormality in schizophrenic patients. Dr. Buchsbaum, in Chapter 2, describes his own work with schizophrenic patients, which has now been extended to larger groups of schizophrenic individuals tested under various experimental conditions. Regional abnormalities of glucose metabolism in other brain areas have also been described in schizophrenic patients, and the relation of these abnormalities to psychiatric symptomatology is described by Drs. Gur and Gur in Chapter 3. Dr. Volkow and her collaborators, in Chapter 4, summarize the current status of the research in schizophrenic patients with FDG and discuss the interpretation of this finding with respect to its clinical significance as well as the specificity and sensitivity of this technique in relation to metabolic defects described in other psychiatric diseases. The use of PET to monitor glucose metabolism was the first clinical application of PET in psychiatric research.

The use of PET in psychiatric research has been expanded to the measurements of regional receptor and enzyme concentrations, neurotransmitter syntheses, and the pharmacokinetics and binding sites of psychoactive drugs. In the late 1960s and early 1970s, groups at BNL; Orsay, France; the University of Kentucky; and McMaster University, Canada, began work on the development of synthetic routes to positron-emitter–labeled radiotracers for probing neurotransmitter metabolism and neurotransmitter receptor properties.

Chemistry has played a central role in the development of PET. In the last two decades, an increasing number of groups worldwide have developed new and interesting ligands for use in research in schizophrenia using PET to provide quantitative information on neuronal activity in a variety of psychotic disorders. Some of the latest work describing these labeled compounds can be found in Chapter 5, by Dr. Schlyer. Most of the work in this area has been devoted to the investigation of abnormalities in the dopamine system occurring in schizophrenic patients. The results of some of these studies have been controversial. Drs. Wong and Young, in Chapter 6, discuss the different methodologies used to attempt to quantitate dopamine receptors in schizophrenic patients and provide comments on discrepancies in results among different groups.

Although PET is a relatively new technique, it has already proven to be able not only to detect brain dysfunction in schizophrenic patients but also to answer some pharmacological questions of clinical relevance. In the second part of Chapter 4, Dr. Volkow and her colleagues discuss some of the findings obtained from PET that have helped solve questions that are of relevance in the treatment of the schizophrenic patient.

PET is an expensive technique, and its utilization in psychiatric diseases has been limited to research in a few centers. Although one can argue that this may limit its usefulness, one can also start to realize that PET is beginning to answer questions that scientists had investigated for decades with much higher research costs and with ambiguous results that could not always be applied to the schizophrenic patient. The feasibility of investigating these questions directly in a living patient cannot be overemphasized. It has been only 10 years since the first investigation of a schizophrenic patient with PET. With improvement in technology and in our methods to measure receptor neurotransmitters and enzymes, we can foresee how PET could advance our knowledge of the etiology and treatment of schizophrenia.

Nora D. Volkow, M.D.
Alfred P. Wolf, Ph.D.

Chapter 1

Positron-Emission Tomography: From the Physics to the Instrument

Bernard Bendriem, Ph.D.

P ositron-emission tomography (PET) is an imaging technique that uses positron emitters to monitor the distribution of radiolabeled tracers and their derivatives in vivo (Brownell et al. 1982; Ter-Pogossian 1977). A wide variety of compounds can be labeled and used to measure biochemical and physiological parameters in the tissue elements such as glucose and oxygen metabolism, protein synthesis, blood flow, receptor densities, and cell division (Fowler and Wolf 1986; Wolf 1981; Wolf and Fowler 1985). A number of applications have emerged for PET in the basic sciences as well as in medicine, including studies of the normal brain and pathological conditions such as tumors, epilepsy, dementia, Parkinson's disease, and psychiatric disorders (Kuhl 1984; Phelps et al. 1982; Volkow et al. 1986, 1988).

A PET experiment involves

1. The production of a positron emitter by a cyclotron or a generator
2. The synthesis of a molecule, containing the radionuclide, that will act as a tracer or as a tracer precursor
3. The external detection of the photons generated by the positron emitter with a "positron camera," with concurrent measurement of the radioactivity in arterial or venous blood
4. The reconstruction of two- or three-dimensional images representing the distribution of the radioactivity in the organ studied
5. The analysis of that distribution through mathematical models based on known chemical and biochemical properties of the tracer and the derivation of physiological parameters

The particulars of each PET experiment will differ depending on

This research was carried out at Brookhaven National Laboratory under Contract No. DE-AC02-76CH00016 from the U.S. Department of Energy and supported by NIH Grant NS-15638.

1

the tracer utilized and to a certain extent on the characteristics of the tomograph.

The most frequent application of PET in the brain has been the measurement of regional glucose metabolism and cerebral blood flow. The methodology to measure the brain glucose metabolism was adapted from the quantitative autoradiographic technique of Sokoloff (Sokoloff et al. 1977). This method uses deoxyglucose (DG), an analogue of glucose, which is labeled with carbon-11 (^{11}C; half-life = 20.4 minutes) or fluorine-18 (^{18}F; half-life = 109.8 minutes). DG is transported bidirectionally across the blood-brain barrier by the same carrier that transports glucose. In the brain, it is phosphorylated similarly to glucose, resulting in the formation of deoxyglucose 6-phosphate (DG-6P). However, at this stage the metabolism of DG stops, unlike that of glucose. After 35 minutes most of the radioactivity is trapped as DG-6P and remains as such for at least 30 minutes. During this period tomographic images are obtained. These images, which reflect the distribution of the positron emitter in the brain, are transformed into metabolic images using a mathematical model that takes into account the concentration of DG in plasma as well as a correction factor that reflects the differences between glucose and DG (Brooks et al. 1987; Huang et al. 1980a; Phelps et al. 1982; Reivich et al. 1979, 1982).

The measurement of regional cerebral blood flow (rCBF) is another widespread application of PET. Several experimental strategies based on the original work of Kety (1951) have been designed to measure rCBF. The most frequently used method involves the intravenous bolus injection of water (H_2O) labeled with oxygen-15 (^{15}O; half-life = 2.07 minutes) (Herscovitch et al. 1983; Raichle et al. 1983). As with other PET tracers, frequent arterial samples are drawn from the time of injection to the end of the scan to measure the concentration of radioactivity in plasma, and a mathematical model is then used to transform the data obtained from the tomograph into values of blood flow. Measurements of CBF and of brain glucose metabolism have been used to monitor regional brain function because of the close association between blood flow, metabolism, and brain activity (Baron et al. 1982; Mazziotta and Phelps 1986; Raichle 1979). Thus, metabolic images obtained reflect the activity occurring in the brain during the initial uptake of DG into the brain (approximately 25–30 minutes), whereas CBF images reflect the activity of the brain over a 30- to 90-second period.

Recently there has been a great interest in using PET to measure receptor densities in the brain. This area will be covered in other chapters in this book.

Physiological and neurochemical values reported by various investigators using PET do not always agree. These values are strongly dependent on the methodology applied (Budinger et al. 1985; Carson 1986; Huang and Phelps 1986; Lammertsma et al. 1987) and on the quantitative abilities of the PET tomograph (Hoffman and Phelps 1986). The effects of different methodologies on quantitative values obtained with PET will be illustrated for the case of receptor measurements in other chapters in this book. In this chapter, I focus on the physical principles of the PET tomograph.

THE APPLIED SCIENCE

History

The idea of using positron emitters to localize brain tumors was suggested by Wrenn et al. (1951) and Brownell and Sweet (1953). The development of transverse cross-sectional imaging of the human body was stimulated by the work of Kuhl and Edwards (1963). The first devices using positron emission were described by Brownell and Sweet (1953), Anger (1967), and Aronow (1967). The first camera using a series of detectors arranged as a ring was built at Brookhaven National Laboratory by Rankowitz et al. (1962) and Robertson et al. (1973). It used 32 thick NaI (sodium iodine) crystals that were arranged to surround the patient. Comprehensive techniques for image reconstruction and their practical implementation on fast computers were developed later (Ter-Pogossian et al. 1975). The algorithms for image reconstruction used in PET are similar to the one used for X-ray computed tomography (CT) and are derived from the work of Cormack (1973) and Hounsfield (1973). Various positron tomographs have been designed, built, and installed in different PET centers, mostly in the United States, Western Europe, and Japan. (For reviews of the development of PET cameras, see Budinger et al. 1979; Jacobson 1988; Kereiakes 1987; Muehllehner and Colsher 1982; Phelps 1977; Ter-Pogossian 1977.) Presently, six companies are commercializing PET cameras (Scanditronix, Hitachi, Shumazdu, CTI-Siemens, Positron Corporation, and UGM Medical Systems). It is anticipated that more companies will join the venture, especially as new clinical applications are developed and the cost of operations is reduced.

Utilization of Positron Emitters

PET utilizes the properties of β+ radioactivity, which is characterized by the emission of positrons from the nucleus of an unstable isotope.

Positron emitters are produced either by a cyclotron (Wolf and Jones 1983) or a chemical generator (Yano 1989).

Three groups of positron emitters can be distinguished. The first group contains oxygen-15 (^{15}O), nitrogen-13 (^{13}N), and carbon-11 (^{11}C) with respective half-lives of 2, 10, and 20.4 minutes. These are isotopes of atoms that are part of most biological structures. They can be used to label molecules without alteration of the original chemical structure. Moreover, their short half-lives minimize radiation exposure to the patient, which allows repeated studies in the same subject in order to assess the stability of the measurement and the effects of interventions. The drawback is that their short half-lives require the presence of a cyclotron on-site for production, and their incorporation into compounds requires the development of rapid methods for organic synthesis.

The second group consists also of cyclotron–produced radionuclides and contains fluorine-18 (^{18}F), bromine-75 (^{75}Br), and bromine-76 (^{76}Br), with half-lives of 1.91, 1.65, and 16 hours, respectively. Their longer half-lives give some flexibility for their transportation from their place of fabrication to their place of utilization. Since in most cases these isotopes are not part of the parent molecule, one must verify that labeling of the molecule does not affect its chemical properties.

The third group comprises radionuclides that can be produced with a generator. The principal radionuclides are rubidium-82 (^{82}Rb), obtained from strontium-82 (^{82}Sr), and gallium-68 (^{68}Ga), obtained from germanium-68 (^{68}Ge). Their use is very attractive but their applications thus far are limited. Copper-62 has been used to label pyruvaldehyde-bis-(N^4-methylthiosemicarbazonato)copper and used successfully to measure CBF (Green et al. 1990).

The Physics of Positron Emission

The positron is a particle with a mass and spin similar to the electron but with an opposite charge. It is emitted by unstable radioelements that possess an excess of protons with regard to their number of neutrons. Indeed, this nuclear reaction is described by the transformation of a proton to a neutron with simultaneous emission of a positron and a neutrino (Evans 1955).

After emission, the positron travels a few millimeters and loses its kinetic energy mainly by successive collisions with electrons. Its maximum range is a function of its maximum kinetic energy, and its average range is about one-third of its maximum range. Table 1-1 details the characteristics of the principal positron emitters used in PET.

Table 1-1. Principal positron emitters used in PET and their main characteristics

Radionuclide	Half-life (minutes)[a]	Number of positrons per disintegration[b]	Mean positron energy[b] (megaelectronvolts)	Path length in water (mm)[c]	Range in water (FWHM) (mm)[c]
^{11}C	20.4	1.00	0.386	1.1	1.1
^{13}N	10.0	1.00	0.492	1.5	1.4
^{15}O	2.1	1.00	0.735	2.7	1.5
^{18}F	109.8	0.97	0.250	0.6	1.0
^{68}Ga	68.2	0.90	0.829	3.1	1.7
^{75}Br	99.0	0.90	0.567[d]	1.9	–
^{76}Br	972.0	0.62	1.200[d]	5.0	–
^{82}Rb	1.25	0.95	1.475	6.6	1.7

[a]From Radiological Health Handbook, U.S. Department of Health, Education, and Welfare, 1970. [b]From Cross et al. 1983. [c]Path length in water of a positron with the mean energy evaluated from Radiological Health Handbook. [d]Assumed to be equal to one-third of the maximum energy. [e]From Cho et al. 1975.

When the positron is almost at rest, a collision with an electron becomes an annihilation reaction and produces the simultaneous emission of two gamma rays, each one with an energy of 511 kiloelectron volts (keV), which are emitted almost 180° apart (De Benedetti et al. 1950). The 511-keV photons travel at nearly the speed of light in human tissues (~ 300,000 km/second or 0.3 mm/picosecond). Since they are emitted simultaneously, the presence of a positron can be assessed by the detection in temporal coincidence of the two 511-keV gamma rays.

Nuclear medicine instrumentation that uses the detection of a single photon as a source of information necessitates a collimator to localize the directions of the incident radiation. The inevitable outcome is a loss of the overall sensitivity of the camera (Budinger et al. 1979). In PET, the collimation is achieved "electronically," as shown in Figure 1-1. If two 511-keV photons are detected within a time

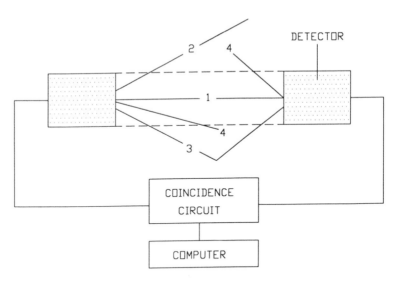

Figure 1-1. Type of events recorded by a PET tomograph. A true event (*1*) is the detection, within the coincidence time, of the two radiations emitted, approximately 180° apart, from a positron source located within the volume of coincidence (outlined by the *dashed lines*). If the positron source is located outside the volume of coincidence, only one radiation can be detected producing a single event (*2*). A scatter event (*3*) is the detection of two radiations, one of which (or both) has undergone a Compton scattering. A random event (*4*) is the detection, in coincidence, of two radiations emitted by two different positron sources.

called the coincidence window (CW), the radioactive source is located somewhere in the volume delineated by the two "coincident" detectors. A source located outside the delineated volume will not be registered. The CW time depends on the characteristics of the detector used and on the difference in distance traveled by the two photons (which in turn depends on the size of the object scanned). It is on the order of 5–20 nanoseconds for most current scanners. Since it is nonnull, so is the probability of detecting, within the CW time, two uncorrelated photons (emitted by two different positrons). The registration of such events, called randoms (Figure 1–1), produces image distortion, and the rate of their occurrence is proportional to the CW time and to the rate of single photons detected by each detector individually (Hoffman et al. 1981). The use of very fast detectors (Allemand et al. 1980; Laval et al. 1983) allows the measurement of the difference between the arrival time of the two photons. This strategy, referred to as time-of-flight (TOF) (Gariod et al. 1982; Mullani et al. 1982; Tomitani 1981), provides some information about the position of the source within the volume of coincidence. The precision of TOF measurement is about 300–1,000 picoseconds. If precision on the order of magnitude of 10 picoseconds (10^{-12} seconds) was achievable, a direct measurement of the tomographic distribution of the radioactive sources would be possible without the need of further processing.

Detection of the 511-keV Photons

A scintillation crystal associated with a photomultiplier (PM) tube is the most frequently used detector in nuclear medicine (Knoll 1979). Every photon is analyzed individually. In the scintillator, it loses all or part of its energy and exchanges it with electrons of the crystal. The crystal radiates this energy as "luminous" photons that, in turn, are going to extract electrons from the photocathode of the PM tube. These photoelectrons are accelerated and directed to a set of dynodes where secondary electrons are created. The overall result is an amplification of the signal in proportion to the amount of energy deposited in the crystal. This signal is then analyzed and digitized electronically.

The Reconstruction Process

Like many other imaging modalities, PET applies the mathematical theory known as "image reconstruction from projections." This technique, derived from the early work of mathematician Radon (1917), has contributed to the revolution of the diagnostic medical field with its application to X-ray computed tomography. Its principle consists in the estimation and representation of a two-dimensional real function F from the measurement of a finite number of its line integrals. In PET, this function represents the amount of positron emitters in a volume element (voxel).

A line integral is a summation of the function F along a given line. In PET the line integral is equal to the number of counts detected by a pair of coincident detectors (which is related to the amount of radioactivity located in the volume intercepted by the two detectors). The set of all line integrals parallel to a given direction is called a projection (Figure 1-2). From the measurement of projections corresponding to directions uniformly sampled from 0 to 180°, it is possible to retrieve the function F.

There are many algorithms possible for this process. The most common is known as the "filtered-back projection." It is easy to implement on a computer, and, if specialized hardware is used, its execution can be very fast (5–20 seconds for a 128×128 matrix). Its main drawback is that it amplifies all the statistical fluctuations associated with the measurement of radioactive process (Alpert et al. 1982; Budinger and Gullberg 1974; Budinger et al. 1977). Iterative

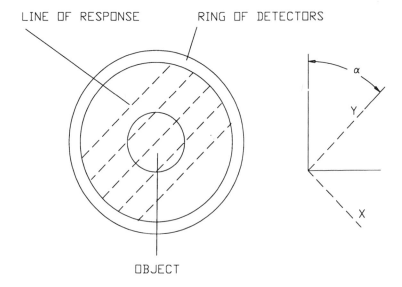

Figure 1-2. Definition of a projection of a given function. A line integral is the summation of the function along a line of response. A line of response is defined by the angle (α) between its direction and a fixed direction and by its distance to the center of the field of view.

techniques that treat the problem as a matrix equation and statistical treatments using the maximum likelihood concept have been extensively studied. They can produce better images; however, the processing time is still too long for routine utilization.

Recently, much interest has been aroused in three-dimensional reconstruction algorithms (Defrise et al. 1988; Rogers et al. 1987; Townsend et al. 1989). Some clinical applications would benefit from a volumetric examination of the brain rather than a tomographic one.

INSTRUMENTATION

Performance

The performance of the PET cameras is of critical importance in order to evaluate the capabilities of the system and to assess the feasibility of performing different types of measurements. I will describe the main variables that influence the performance of PET cameras.

Resolution. The resolution of the imaging device characterizes its ability to detect and quantitate positron sources in various structures. In principle, a structure that has the same dimension as the resolution of the instrument can be delineated on the image. However, to obtain accurate quantitation of the amount of radioactivity within a structure, its dimensions have to be at least twice the resolution of the instrument (Hoffman et al. 1979). The resolution of PET cameras has improved from 2 cm to 0.5 cm in the last decade. A system developed at the University of California, Berkeley, and described recently (Derenzo et al. 1988) has been built with 2.6-mm resolution, approaching the limits imposed by the travel of the positron in tissue and by the physics of coincidence detection.

The path length of a positron (distance traveled by the positron before it annihilates with an electron) is of the order of 1 to several millimeters depending on the radionuclide. However, since it follows a tortuous path, its range, or penetration depth, is usually smaller. Important positron ranges have been measured by Cho et al. (1975). Table 1–1 provides the main characteristics of the current positron emitters. Fluorine-18 has the smallest positron range and is thus best suited for high-resolution tomography.

Another limiting factor is the fact that the emission of the two 511-keV radiations is not strictly 180° apart (the two rays deviate from colinearity with a full-width half maximum [FWHM] of 0.5°). As a consequence, an error in the localization of the positron is introduced. This error increases with the distance between the two coincident detectors (~2 mm [FWHM] for a 100-cm separation between detectors).

There are different types of resolution in a PET system:

1. The *intrinsic resolution* refers to the resolution of the individual detector pair.
2. The *image resolution* is the practical resolution of the system and is dependent on the intrinsic resolution and on the processing necessary to produce the image (Huang et al. 1980b; Rowland 1979).
3. The *axial resolution* refers to the slice thickness. Most PET cameras (those called multislice PET systems) have a nonuniform axial resolution (Hoffman et al. 1982).

Resolution is best when measured at the center of the field of view (FOV) of the imaging device.

Sensitivity. The sensitivity of a PET scanner provides information about the number of counts available to produce an image for a given source of radioactivity. It is usually measured by the number of counts detected by the tomograph when a cylinder of 20 cm in diameter containing a radioactive source with a specific activity of 1 μCi/cc (3.7×10^4 Bq/cc) is scanned. The size of the cylinder is chosen to emulate a head-scanning situation. The number of counts available is a function of the object scanned; in particular, it is strongly dependent on the auto-attenuation of the radiation in the object. For instance, in the case of a 20-cm cylinder filled with water, only 18% of the pairs of photons will escape without interacting with the water. In a 13-cm phantom (emulating a baboon-head situation), this number becomes 32%.

For current PET cameras, the sensitivity number ranges from 3,000–30,000 counts per second and per tomographic slice as defined above. The sensitivity of the camera is dependent on the intrinsic efficiency of each individual detector (ratio of the number of counts detected over the number of photons that have actually reached an individual detector) and on the geometry of the detection system (solid angle). The sensitivity should consider only the number of true coincidences recorded, and the random and scattered radiations should be subtracted from the sensitivity number. Scattered radiation represents events that have deviated from their original path due to interactions. Variables in the PET camera that influence the number of random and scattered radiations include the diameter of the detection system, the length and type of inter-ring septa used in a multi-ring camera, and the energy thresholds at which the system is operated (Tanaka et al. 1982). Random and scattered radiation increases with a larger distance between septa and decreases with a larger diameter of the ring and with higher energy thresholds (Derenzo 1980).

Dead-time. Dead-time represents the time during which the system cannot process data and implies a maximum number of data that can be handled per unit of time. The dead-time of a system is a very complex parameter. It is different for each type of detector and strongly affected by the design of the electronics that process the data. It is related to the total number of counts that are analyzed, whether they are single, random, scattered, or multiples. It is therefore very important to minimize all undesirable photons in order to process only those carrying useful information.

Critical to the accuracy of the final result is the way the PET systems handle and correct for these events. This will be detailed further.

Detection System

Geometry. Although some systems are designed to directly produce volumetric data (Burnham et al. 1988; Muehllehner et al. 1988), most PET cameras are designed to organize the data in tomographic slices. The detection system surrounds the object, and the most common geometry configurations are the circular and the hexagonal ones. The circular geometry has the advantage of covering and scanning all of the object. Its drawback is that the solid angle of detection varies with the position of the source and must be corrected by software. Furthermore, the resolution achieved with circular ring detectors is not uniform along the FOV due to crystal penetration when the photon enters the crystal with a nonnormal incidence (Wong et al. 1984). This effect has been the object of recent investigation, and some correction schemes have been proposed (Huessman et al. 1989).

The hexagonal geometry produces a more uniform response. However, for some angles of projection, the sensitivity drops, producing an area of "missing data." This requires the use of algorithms developed for image reconstruction from "missing projections" (Ollinger and Karp 1988).

Different motions of the detection system have been proposed and used to improve sampling and to cover the gap that exists between two adjacent crystals. Among them are the wobbling motion (circular translation) (Bohm et al. 1978; Ter-Pogossian et al. 1978) and the clam shell motion. The actual tendency, however, is to build stationary machines (to reduce the complexity of the engineering aspect) using very small crystals (Muehllehner and Karp 1988; Tanaka 1987).

Detectors. Different types of scintillation crystals have been employed as detectors in PET. A good scintillator must have a high linear attenuation coefficient (capacity of absorbing all the energy of the photons), a good light yield in the maximum sensitivity range of the phototube (number of "luminous" photons created), and a fast scintillation decay (time necessary for the light to be emitted). In addition, it should be nonhygroscopic, removing the necessity for encapsulation. Table 1-2 shows the principal characteristics of the crystals used in PET.

Bismuth germanate (BGO) is the most commonly used crystal because of its high stopping power, which makes possible the utilization of small crystals to achieve high spatial resolution (Cho and Faruhki 1977). The main drawback of BGO is its relatively slow scintillation decay and its poor light yield (compared with NaI). This leads to important intrinsic dead-time and requires the use of a large CW (Derenzo 1981).

Cesium fluoride (CsF) was introduced to overcome this aspect. It allows fast dynamic scans at high count rates (Allemand et al. 1980). It has a very small decay constant. With this crystal the CW necessary to achieve good detection of coincident photons is on the order of 5–10 nanoseconds and is less than that of BGO (12–20 nanoseconds). Its major drawback is that it is hygroscopic and needs to be encapsulated, making it difficult to achieve very high spatial resolution using this crystal.

Barium fluoride (BaF_2) is a fast crystal, like CsF, yet it is a denser crystal and is not hygroscopic. However, it is considerably more expensive. Both crystals have poor energy resolution, and their energy threshold must be set around 150 keV to preserve their efficiency (Wong 1988).

As previously described, a crystal scintillator coupled with a PM tube is the most common type of detector used. The association of the crystal with the PM tube can consist of one PM tube per crystal, one PM tube per several crystals, or many PM tubes coupled to a large crystal. The use of one PM tube per crystal requires the crystals to be isolated with interdetector septa to prevent photon crossover. These

Table 1-2.   Crystal scintillators used in PET and their main characteristics

Scintillator	Density	Decay constant (nanoseconds)	Light output (% of NaI)
NaI (Tl)	3.67	230	100
BGO	7.13	350	8
CsF	6.61	5	4
BaF_2	6.89	0.6 and 620	10

septa reduce the overall sensitivity of the system. Moveover, the intrinsic resolution is, in that case, limited by the practical size of the available PM tube. In a large crystal coupled with many PM tubes, an event is localized from the relative output of the different PM tubes (Karp et al. 1986). Such a system can achieve high resolution in all dimensions (in the tomographic plane as well as in the axial direction) and is well suited for real three-dimensional reconstruction. Without specialized electronics and adequate pulse shaping, it will suffer, however, from a large dead-time due to the time necessary to analyze the light from all PM tubes (Mankoff et al. 1989; Yamamoto et al. 1989). Hybrid detectors called blocs have been proposed (Casey and Nutt 1986; Erikson et al. 1987). They consist of a number of crystals arranged in a bloc of crystals (8–64) coupled to a small number of PM tubes (2–4). Another possible approach is the use of light guides to couple several small crystals to a few PM tubes (Wong et al. 1987; Yamamoto et al. 1986a).

DATA PROCESSING AND IMAGE QUALITY

Correction of Raw Data

The raw data obtained from the PET detectors must be processed before they are fed to the reconstruction algorithms. I will describe the correction steps in the order in which they are most frequently performed.

Random correction. Random coincidences consist of the simultaneous detection of two uncorrelated photons and lead to mispositioning of positron sources with a consequent blurring of the image (Hoffman et al. 1981). Since their number increases as the square of the radioactivity in the object, they are particularly problematic when doing studies with high levels of activity such as the measurement of blood flow after injection of greater than 50 mCi of labeled water. Random counts should be subtracted from the total number of counts obtained. There are different ways to estimate the number of randoms. One can measure them by counting the number of coincidences detected after a certain delay has been introduced in the coincidence circuit. If the delay is long enough (at least 16 nanoseconds), then all coincidences registered can only be random. Another technique evaluates the number of randoms from the measurement of a single count rate for each detector. In effect, if detector 1 measures N_1 singles per second and detector 2 measures N_2 singles per second, the random rate registered by the detector pair is given by $N_1 \times N_2 \times T$, where T is the CW value. A third technique consists of subtracting a constant level from the projection data. This technique is the least accurate because it assumes that the randoms are uniformly distributed (which is only true for a relatively symmetrical distribution of radioactivity).

Detection linearity and uniformity. The correction for detection linearity is mainly the correction for the dead-time of the detector. The fraction of events lost increases with the rate of events detected. Hence it can become problematic when doing studies that require injection of high doses of radioactivity. The consequence of dead-time is an underestimation of the level of radioactivity (Mazoyer et al. 1985; Thompson and Meyer 1987). Different techniques have been proposed (Germano and Hoffman 1988; Yamamoto et al. 1986b) to correct for dead-time losses that are based on the measurement of randoms and/or multiples (detection of three photons or more within the CW). However, these corrections work up to a certain value of the count rate and there is a limitation on the amount of data that a positron camera can handle. One must assess it by adequate phantom measurements.

The nonuniformity of detection has two origins: the first one is geometrical, and the second one is due to intrinsic variation of efficiency of individual detectors. The way to take into account these variations is to measure them using a perfectly uniform phantom (Hoffman et al. 1989).

Correction for scattered radiations. This is probably the most complex to perform, and, as a matter of fact, it is not done systematically. The fraction of scattered radiation depends on the detection system design, the radioactive source distribution, and the scattering medium. Compton scattering is the most frequent type of interaction for 511-keV photons in the human body. When a photon undergoes such an interaction it loses part of its energy. However, the energy of scattered photons that escape the human body has a range of 400–500 keV and is very difficult to discriminate from the energy of unscattered radiation due to the limited energy resolution of the detectors.

Correction schemes have been proposed that are based on the observed distribution of the scattered radiation measured experimentally. This type of correction assumes a uniform scattering medium and provides a good first-order correction for brain scans (Bendriem et al. 1986; Bergstrom et al. 1983).

Correction for auto-attenuation. The correction for auto-attenuation has a theoretical solution in PET. It can be measured with a source located outside the object to be scanned. A reference scan is obtained without the object, followed by a scan with the object in position. The procedure is similar to an X-ray CT scan. For each detector pair, the ratio between the two measurements provides the correction factor for attenuation (Huang et al. 1979).

Image Accuracy

In the following section I emphasize the sources of error attached to PET measurements.

Noise in the image. Noise in the image from radioactive fluctuations has its origin in the Poissonian nature of radioactive emission and detection. These fluctuations are inversely related to the square root of the total number of true counts detected. The fluctuations are not distributed uniformly in a given image. They are dependent on the distribution of the radioactivity and on the attenuation media surrounding the sources (Budinger et al. 1977).

In general, all the statistical fluctuations are exacerbated by the different correction steps. Propagation of noise varies like the square of each correction factor. It is, then, important to keep them close to unity.

There are other parameters that will affect the quality of the images such as length of scan and choice of a reconstruction filter. The longer the scan the greater the number of counts detected. However, there is a trade-off between the quality of the image obtained and the time sequence that will allow one to observe dynamic processes (Mazoyer et al. 1986). There is also a trade-off between image quality and image resolution from the reconstruction filter (Tanaka and Iiuma 1975) (Figure 1-3).

Effects of limited resolution. An important limiting factor in PET is the partial volume effect. It refers to the inaccuracy in quantitation of structures that are smaller than two times the image resolution in all directions (Mazziotta et al. 1981). In most PET cameras, the resolution (axial as well as transverse) is not uniform along the FOV. Partial volume effect is then dependent on the source position, and its correction is a delicate process (Bendriem et al. 1989). It has been assessed by phantom experiments (e.g., a cylinder with a diameter of one times the resolution will undergo a quantitation loss by a factor of two). However, phantom experiments simulate only ideal situations, simplified with regard to the complexity of anatomy (especially brain anatomy). An anatomical image (provided by a magnetic resonance image [MRI] or an X-ray CT scan) may be beneficial in order to localize specific structures and measure their dimensions. Superimposition of an anatomical image into the PET requires a very precise definition of landmark points to locate the level at which the scans were taken on both imaging modalities. Several strategies have been proposed to give precise alignment of these two imaging modalities (Pelizzari et al. 1989; Wilson and Mountz 1989).

The motion of the subject during the scan can increase the blurring of the image. It is therefore desirable to have adequate immobilization of the subject during the scan. A number of head holders have been proposed for this purpose and are currently being used (Kearfott et al. 1984). These head holders must also allow adequate repositioning when a subject is taken in and out of the camera. Important parameters in the design of head holders include their immobilization capacity, degree of comfort, adequacy for repositioning, and the time

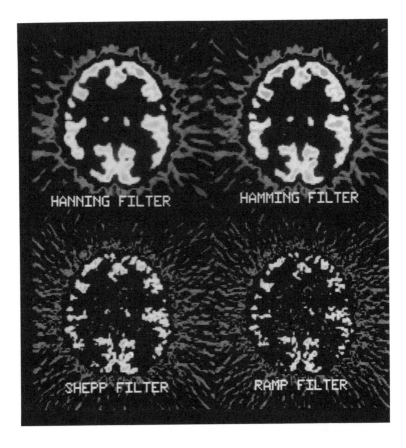

Figure 1-3. Fluorodeoxyglucose images reconstructed with different filters. The image resolution is dependent on the type of filter used.

necessary to build them (in most cases they are made on demand prior to the scan).

In most circumstances, two adjacent structures, containing two different activity levels, can hardly be completely isolated due to the blurring that each one induces in the other. The analysis of images is then a delicate task easily subject to systematic errors. To alleviate subjectivity in the definition of the structure of interest, a number of techniques for automatic definition of the anatomical region have been derived (Evans et al. 1988; Fox et al. 1985). One has to be certain, however, that they are bias-free, reproducible, and accurate. In any case, the range of error associated with the mode of definition used (manual versus automatic) as well as the partial volume effect should be assessed for each scanner and each type of study and included in subsequent analysis (Mazziotta and Koslow 1987).

BRAIN IMAGING

I have reviewed the potential sources of error and some solutions to eliminate (or at least minimize) their effects on the accuracy of PET data. It is important, when choosing a PET camera, to assess its performance and its ability to handle the different correction steps, with regard to the type of study considered.

Brain imaging, for example, requires higher resolution than other organs, due to the complexity in size and shape of the brain structures. As mentioned earlier, accurate measurement of the activity concentration is only possible for structures that are at least two times the image resolution of the positron camera in all directions (transverse as well as axial). Quantitation of smaller structures will be dependent on many factors, such as contrast with surrounding tissues and size and shape of the region of interest chosen. Ignorance of these effects will provide erroneous measurements and can lead to misinterpretation of data.

In static brain imaging, such as ^{18}F-labeled fluorodeoxyglucose scanning, errors due to photon statistics, dead-time losses, and randoms are minimized due to the combination of two factors: the activity injected is low and the rate of acquisition of data is low. Since the count rate is relatively constant 35 minutes after injection, it is possible to acquire data for at least 20 minutes. On most PET cameras, the number of events collected is, in that case, sufficient to produce high-quality images.

Dynamic imaging, using short half-life isotopes such as ^{15}O, requires the injection of a high bolus of radioactivity. In these situations the count rate of the PET camera varies with time, and issues such as dead-time losses and randoms become a source of error. When evaluating the kinetics of a tracer in the brain, imaging times can be very short (on the order of 10 seconds), which leads to images with very few counts and hence with poor statistical quality. Because of these issues, the limitations and capabilities of the particular PET instrument utilized need to be considered before designing an experimental protocol.

FUTURE DIRECTIONS FOR PET TECHNOLOGY

At this stage, the only 3-mm resolution (FWHM) tomograph is a single-ring tomograph. Research is in progress to build a multi-ring system with this level of resolution.

It is expected that future improvements of detector design will lead to better overall sensitivity without loss of resolution. Such improvements will be achieved if better timing performance of a tomograph using BGO crystals or better spatial and energy resolution of a tomograph using BaF_2 crystals can be obtained.

It is also expected that efforts will be made in the design of instruments capable of producing direct volumetric information.

These issues must be worked out in order to increase the accuracy of the PET scanner and to allow a better interpretation and understanding of PET images.

REFERENCES

Allemand R, Gresset C, Vacher J: Potential advantages of a cesium fluoride scintillator for a time of flight positron camera. J Nucl Med 21:153–155, 1980

Alpert NM, Chesler DA, Correia JA, et al: Estimation of the local statistical noise in emission computed tomography. IEEE Transactions in Medical Imaging 1:142–146, 1982

Anger HO: Radioisotope cameras, in Instrumentation in Nuclear Medicine, Vol 1. New York, Academic, 1967, pp 485–552

Aronow S: Positron scanning, in Instrumentation in Nuclear Medicine, Vol 1. New York, Academic, 1967, pp 461–483

Baron JC, Lebrun-Grandie P, Collard P, et al: Noninvasive measurement of blood flow, oxygen consumption, and glucose utilization in the same brain regions in man by positron emission tomography: concise communication. J Nucl Med 23:391–399, 1982

Bendriem B, Soussaline F, Compagnolo R, et al: A technique for the correction of scattered radiation in a PET system using time-of-flight information. J Comput Assist Tomogr 10:287–295, 1986

Bendriem B, Christman DR, Schlyer DJ: Dependence of the recovery coefficient in multislice positron emission tomography. J Nucl Med 30:893, 1989

Bergstrom M, Eriksson L, Bohm C, et al: Correction for scattered radiation in a ring detector positron camera by integral transformation of the projection. J Comput Assist Tomogr 7:42–50, 1983

Bohm C, Eriksson L, Bergstrom M, et al: A computer assisted ring detector positron camera system for reconstruction tomography of the brain. IEEE Transactions in Nuclear Sciences 25:624–637, 1978

Brooks R, Hatazawa J, Di Chiro G, et al: Human cerebral glucose metabolism determined by positron emission tomography: a revisit. J Cereb Blood Flow Metab 7:427–432, 1987

Brownell GL, Sweet WH: Localization of brain tumors with positron emitters. Nucleonics 11:40–45, 1953

Brownell GL, Budinger TF, Lauterbur PC, et al: Positron tomography and nuclear magnetic resonance imaging. Science 215:619–626, 1982

Budinger TF, Gullberg GT: Three-dimensional reconstruction in nuclear medicine emission imaging. IEEE Transactions in Nuclear Sciences 21:2–20, 1974

Budinger TF, Derenzo SE, Gullberg GT, et al: Emission computed assisted tomography with single photon and positron annihilation photon emitters. J Comput Assist Tomogr 1:131–145, 1977

Budinger TF, Gullberg GT, Huesman RH: Emission computed tomography, in Image Reconstruction From Projections: Implementation and Application. Edited by Herman GT. New York, Springer-Verlag, 1979, pp 147–246

Budinger TF, Huesman RH, Knittel B, et al: Physiological modeling of dynamic measurements of metabolism using positron emission tomography, in The Metabolism of the Human Brain Studied With Positron Emission Tomography. Edited by Greitz T. New York, Raven, 1985, pp 165–183

Burnham C, Bradshaw J, Kaufman D, et al: A positron tomograph employing a one dimension BGO scintillation camera. IEEE Transactions in Nuclear Sciences 30:661–664, 1983

Burnham CA, Kaufman DE, Chesler DA, et al: Cylindrical PET detector design. IEEE Transactions in Nuclear Sciences 35:675–679, 1988

Carson RE: Parameter estimation in positron emission tomography, in Positron Emission Tomography and Autoradiography: Principles and Applications for the Brain and Heart. Edited by Phelps M, Mazziotta J, Schelbert H. New York, Raven, 1986, pp 347–390

Casey ME, Nutt R: A multicrystal two dimensional BGO detector system for positron emission tomography. IEEE Transactions in Nuclear Sciences 33:460–463, 1986

Cho ZH, Faruhki MR: Bismuth germanate as a potential scintillation detector in positron cameras. J Nucl Med 18:840–844, 1977

Cho ZH, Chan JK, Eriksson L, et al: Positron ranges obtained from biomedically important positron-emitting radionuclides. J Nucl Med 16:1174–1176, 1975

Cormack AM: Reconstruction of densities from their projections with application in radiological physics. Phys Med Biol 18:195–207, 1973

Cross WG, Ing H, Freedman N: A short atlas of beta-ray spectra. Phys Med Biol 28:1251–1260, 1983

De Benedetti SC, Owen WR, Konoker C, et al: On the angular distribution of two-photon annihilation radiation. Physiol Rev 77:205–212, 1950

Defrise M, Kuijk S, Deconinck F: A new three-dimensional reconstruction for positron cameras using plane detectors. Phys Med Biol 33:34–51, 1988

Derenzo SE: Method for optimizing side shielding in positron emission tomography and for comparing detector materials. J Nucl Med 21:971–977, 1980

Derenzo SE: Monte Carlo calculations of the detection efficiency of arrays of NaI(TI), BGO, CsF, Ge, and plastic detectors for 511 keV photons. IEEE Transactions in Nuclear Sciences 28:131–136, 1981

Derenzo SE, Huesman RH, Cahoon JL, et al: A positron tomograph with 600 BGO crystals and 2.6 mm resolution. IEEE Transactions in Nuclear Sciences 35:659–664, 1988

Eriksson L, Bohm C, Kesselberg M, et al: Design studies of two possible detector blocks for high resolution positron emission tomography of the brain. IEEE Transactions in Nuclear Sciences 34:344–348, 1987

Evans AC, Beil C, Marrett S, et al: Anatomical-functional correlation using an adjustable MRI–based region of interest atlas with positron emission tomography. J Cereb Blood Flow Metab 8:513–530, 1988

Evans RD: The Atomic Nucleus. New York, McGraw-Hill, 1955

Fowler JS, Wolf AP: Positron emitter-labeled compounds: priorities and problems, in Positron Emission Tomography and Autoradiography: Principles and Applications for the Brain and Heart. Edited by Phelps M, Mazziotta J, Schelbert H. New York, Raven, 1986, pp 391–450

Fox PT, Perlmutter JS, Raichle ME: A stereotactic method of anatomical localization for positron emission tomography. J Comput Assist Tomogr 9:141–153, 1985

Gariod R, Allemand R, Cormoreche E, et al: The LETI positron tomograph architecture and time-of-flight improvements, in Proceedings of Workshop on Time-of-Flight Tomography. Saint Louis, MO, IEEE, 1982, pp 25–29

Germano G, Hoffman EJ: Investigation of count rate and deadtime characteristics of a high resolution PET system. J Comput Assist Tomogr 12:836–846, 1988

Green MA, Mathias CJ, Welch MJ, et al: Copper-62 labeled pyruvaldehyde bis (N^4 methylthiosemicarbazonato)copper (11): synthesis and evaluation as a positron emission tracer for cerebral and myocardial perfusion. J Nucl Med 31:1989–1996, 1990

Herscovitch P, Markham J, Raichle ME: Brain blood flow measured with intravenous $H_2 15O$, I: theory and error analysis. J Nucl Med 24:782–789, 1983

Hoffman EJ, Phelps ME: Positron emission tomography: principles and quantitation, in Positron Emission Tomography and Autoradiography: Principles and Applications for the Brain and Heart. Edited by Phelps M, Mazziotta J, Schelbert H. New York, Raven, 1986, pp 237–286

Hoffman EJ, Huang SC, Phelps ME: Quantitation in positron emission computed tomography, 1: effect of object size. J Comput Assist Tomogr 3:299–308, 1979

Hoffman EJ, Huang SC, Phelps ME, et al: Quantitation in positron emission tomography, 4: effect of accidental coincidences. J Comput Assist Tomogr 5:391–400, 1981

Hoffman EJ, Huang SC, Plummer D, et al: Quantitation in positron emission computed tomography, 6: effect of nonuniform resolution. J Comput Assist Tomogr 6:987–999, 1982

Hoffman EJ, Guerrero TM, Germano G: PET system calibrations and corrections for quantitative and spatially accurate images. IEEE Transactions in Nuclear Sciences 36:1108–1112, 1989

Hounsfield GN: Computerized transverse axial scanning (tomography), part I: description of the system. Br J Radiol 46:1016–1022, 1973

Huang SC, Phelps ME: Principles of tracer kinetic modeling in positron emission tomography and autoradiography, in Positron Emission Tomography and Autoradiography: Principles and Applications for the Brain and Heart. Edited by Phelps M, Mazziotta J, Schelbert H. New York, Raven, 1986, pp 287–346

Huang SC, Hoffman EJ, Phelps ME: Quantitation in positron emission computed tomography, 2: effects of inaccurate attenuation correction. J Comput Assist Tomogr 3:804–814, 1979

Huang SC, Phelps ME, Hoffman EJ, et al: Noninvasive determination of local cerebral metabolic rate of glucose in man. Am J Physiol 238:E69–E82, 1980a

Huang SC, Hoffman EJ, Phelps ME: Quantitation in positron emission computed tomography, 3: effect of sampling. J Comput Assist Tomogr 4:819–826, 1980b

Huesman RH, Salmeron EM, Baker JR: Compensation for crystal penetration in high resolution positron tomography. IEEE Transactions in Nuclear Sciences 36:1100–1107, 1989

Jacobson HG: Instrumentation in positron emission tomography. JAMA 259:1531–1536, 1988

Karp JS, Muehllehner G, Beerbohm D, et al: Event localization in a continuous scintillation detector using digital processing. IEEE Transactions in Nuclear Sciences 33:550–555, 1986

Kearfott KJ, Rottenberg DA, Knowles RJR: A new headholder for PET, CT, and NMR imaging. J Comput Assist Tomogr 8:1217–1220, 1984

Kereiakes JG: The history and development of medical physics instrumentation: nuclear medicine. Med Phys 14:146–155, 1987

Kety SS: The theory and applications of the exchange of inert gas at the lungs and tissues. Pharmacol Rev 3:1–41, 1951

Knoll GF: Radiation Detection and Measurement. New York, John Wiley, 1979

Kuhl DE: Imaging local brain function with emission computed tomography. Radiology 150:625–631, 1984

Kuhl DE, Edwards RQ: Image separation radioisotope scanning. Radiology 80:653–661, 1963

Kuhl DE, Wagner H, Alavi A, et al: Positron emission tomography: clinical status in the United States in 1987. J Nucl Med 29:1136–1143, 1988

Lammertsma AA, Brooks DJ, Frackowiak SJ, et al: Measurement of glucose utilisation with [^{18}F]2-fluoro-2-deoxy-D-glucose: a comparison of different analytical methods. J Cereb Blood Flow Metab 7:161–172, 1987

Laval M, Moszynski M, Allemand R, et al: Barium fluoride—inorganic scintillator for subnanosecond timing. Nuclear Instruments and Methods 206:169–176, 1983

Mankoff DA, Muehllehner G, Karp JS: The high count rate performance of a two-dimensionally positron-sensitive detector for positron emission tomography. Phys Med Biol 34:437–456, 1989

Mazoyer BM, Roos MS, Huesman RH: Dead time correction and counting statistics for positron tomography. Phys Med Biol 30:385–399, 1985

Mazoyer BM, Huesman RH, Budinger TF, et al: Dynamic PET data analysis. J Comput Assist Tomogr 10:645–653, 1986

Mazziotta JC, Koslow SH: Assessment of goals and obstacles in data acquisition and analysis from emission tomography: report of a series of international workshops. J Cereb Blood Flow Metab 7:S1–S31, 1987

Mazziotta JC, Phelps ME: Positron emission tomography studies of the brain, in Positron Emission Tomography and Autoradiography: Principles and Applications for the Brain and Heart. Edited by Phelps ME, Mazziotta JC, Schelbert H. New York, Raven, 1986, pp 493–580

Mazziotta JC, Phelps ME, Plummer D, et al: Quantitation in positron emission computed tomography, 5: physical—anatomical effects. J Comput Assist Tomogr 5:734–743, 1981

Muehllehner G, Colsher JG: Instrumentation, in Computed Emission Tomography. Edited by Ell PJ, Holman BL. Oxford, Oxford University Press, 1982, pp 3–41

Muehllehner G, Karp JS: Advances in SPECT and PET. IEEE Transactions in Nuclear Sciences 35:639–643, 1988

Muehllehner G, Karp JS, Mankoff DA, et al: Design and performance of a new positron tomograph. IEEE Transactions in Nuclear Sciences 35:670–674, 1988

Mullani NA, Wong WH, Hartz RK: Design of Tofpet: a high resolution time-of-flight positron camera, in Proceedings of Workshop on Time-of-Flight Tomography. Saint Louis, MO, IEEE, 1982, pp 31–36

Ollinger JM, Karp JS: An evaluation of three algorithms for reconstructing images from data with missing projections. IEEE Transactions in Nuclear Sciences 35:629–634, 1988

Pelizzari CA, Chen GTY, Spelbring DR, et al: Accurate three-dimensional registration of CT, PET, and/or MR images of the brain. J Comput Assist Tomogr 13:20–26, 1989

Phelps ME: Emission computed tomography. Semin Nucl Med 7:337–365, 1977

Phelps ME, Huang SC, Hoffman EJ, et al: Tomographic measurements of local cerebral glucose metabolic rate in humans with (F^{18}) 2-fluoro-2-deoxy-D-glucose: validation of method. Ann Neurol 6:371–388, 1979

Phelps ME, Mazziotta JC, Huang SC: Study of cerebral function with positron computed tomography. J Cereb Blood Flow Metab 2:113–162, 1982

Radon J: Ueber die Bestimmung von Funktionen durch ihre Interrahwerte laengs gewisser Mannifgfaltigkciten. Math Phys 69:262–271, 1917

Raichle ME: Quantitative in vivo autoradiography with positron emission tomography. Brain Res 1:47–68, 1979

Raichle ME, Martin RW, Herscovitch P, et al: Brain blood flow measured with intravenous $H_2^{15}O$, II: implementation and validation. J Nucl Med 24:790–798, 1983

Rankowitz S, Robertson JS, Higinbotham WA, et al: Positron scanner for locating brain tumors, in IRE International Convention Record, Part 9. 1962, pp 49–56

Reivich M, Kuhl D, Wolf A, et al: The $[^{18}F]$-fluorodeoxy glucose method for the measurement of local cerebral glucose in man. Circ Res 44:127–137, 1979

Reivich M, Alavi A, Wolf A, et al: Use of 2-deoxy-D$[1-^{11}C]$-glucose for the determination of local cerebral glucose metabolism in humans: variations within and between subjects. J Cereb Blood Flow Metab 2:307–319, 1982

Robertson JS, Marr RB, Rosenblum M, et al: 32-Crystal positron transverse section detector, in Tomographic Imaging in Nuclear Medicine. Edited by Freedman GS. New York, Springer-Verlag, 1973, pp 142–153

Rogers JG, Harrop R, Kinahan PE: The theory of three-dimensional image reconstruction for PET. IEEE Transactions on Medical Imaging 6:239–243, 1987

Rowland SW: Computer implementation of image reconstruction formulas, in Image Reconstruction From Projections: Implementation and Application. Edited by Herman GT. New York, Springer-Verlag, 1979, pp 9–80

Sokoloff L, Reivich M, Kennedy C, et al: The $[^{14}C]$deoxyglucose method for the measurement of local cerebral glucose utilization: theory, procedure, and normal values in the conscious and anesthetized albino rat. J Neurochem 28:897–916, 1977

Tanaka E: Recent progress on single photon and positron emission tomography—from detectors to algorithms. IEEE Transactions in Nuclear Sciences 34:313–320, 1987

Tanaka E, Iiuma TA: Correction functions for optimizing the reconstructed image in transverse section scan. Phys Med Biol 20:789–798, 1975

Tanaka E, Nohara N, Tomitani T, et al: Analytical study of the performance of a multilayer positron computed tomography scanner. J Comput Assist Tomogr 6:350–364, 1982

Ter-Pogossian MM: Basic principles of computed axial tomography. Semin Nucl Med 7:109–127, 1977

Ter-Pogossian MM, Phelps ME, Hoffman EJ, et al: A positron-emission transaxial tomograph for nuclear imaging (PETT). Radiology 114:89–98, 1975

Ter-Pogossian MM, Mullani NA, Hood JT, et al: Design consideration for a positron emission transverse tomograph (PETT V) for imaging the brain. J Comput Assist Tomogr 2:539–544, 1978

Thompson CJ, Meyer E: The effect of live time in components of a positron tomograph on image quantification. IEEE Transactions in Nuclear Sciences 34:337–343, 1987

Tomitani T: Image reconstruction and noise evaluation in photon time-of-flight assisted positron emission tomography. IEEE Transactions in Nuclear Sciences 28:4582–4589, 1981

Townsend DW, Spinks T, Jones T, et al: Three dimensional reconstruction of PET data from a multi-ring camera. IEEE Transactions in Nuclear Sciences 36:1056–1065, 1989

Volkow ND, Brodie JD, Wolf AP, et al: Brain organization in schizophrenia. J Cereb Blood Flow Metab 6:441–446, 1986

Volkow ND, Mullani NA, Bendriem B: Positron emission tomography instrumentation: an overview. American Journal of Physiological Imaging 3:142–153, 1988

Wilson NW, Mountz JM: A reference system for neuroanatomical localization on functional reconstructed cerebral images. J Comput Assist Tomogr 13:174–178, 1989

Wolf AP: Special characteristics and potential for radiopharmaceuticals for positron emission tomography. Semin Nucl Med 11:2–11, 1981

Wolf AP, Fowler JS: Positron emitter-labeled radiotracers: chemical considerations, in Positron Emission Tomography. Edited by Reivich M, Alavi A. New York, Alan R Liss, 1985, pp 63–80

Wolf AP, Jones WB: Cyclotrons for biomedical radioisotope production. Radiochimica Acta 34:1–7, 1983

Wong WH: PET camera performance design evaluation for BGO and BaF_2 scintillators (non-time-of-flight). J Nucl Med 29:338–347, 1988

Wong WH, Mullani NA, Wardworth G, et al: Characteristics of small barium fluoride (BaF^2) scintillator for high intrinsic resolution time-of-flight positron emission tomography. IEEE Transactions in Nuclear Sciences 31:381–386, 1984

Wong WH, Jing M, Bendriem B, et al: A slanting light-guide analog decoding high resolution detector for positron emission tomography camera. IEEE Transactions in Nuclear Sciences 34:280–284, 1987

Wrenn FW, Good ML, Handler P: The use of positron emitting radioisotopes for the localization of brain tumors. Science 113:525–532, 1951

Yamamoto S, Miura S, Iida H, et al: A BGO detector unit for a stationary high resolution PET. J Comput Assist Tomogr 10:851–855, 1986a

Yamamoto S, Masaharu A, Shuichi M, et al: Deadtime correction method using random coincidence for PET. J Nucl Med 27:1925–1928, 1986b

Yamamoto S, Iida H, Amano M, et al: Count rate capability considerations and results for a positron emission tomograph. IEEE Transactions in Nuclear Sciences 35:1020–1024, 1989

Yano Y: Radioisotope generator for short-lived positron emitters applicable to positron emission tomography. Nuclear Instruments and Methods in Physics Research B40-B41:1105–1109, 1989

Chapter 2

Positron-Emission Tomography and Regional Brain Metabolism in Schizophrenia Research

Monte S. Buchsbaum, M.D.

W here in the brain are the defects associated with schizophrenia localized? The widespread involvement of behavior and
cognitive function seen in schizophrenic patients has made it very
difficult to localize the brain pathology in these individuals. Traditional methods of gross examination of the brain at autopsy and
microscopic sections of selected areas have not yielded a definitive
answer to this question. Positron-emission tomography (PET), with
its ability to provide functional images of brain metabolism in vivo,
provides a methodology to address cerebral localization of functional
deficits in schizophrenia.

Pioneering studies of human brain metabolism in schizophrenia
using the method of oxygen arteriovenous difference were made by
Himwich et al. (1939) and Wortis et al. (1940–41). These studies
revealed no differences between normal individuals and never-medicated schizophrenic patients in whole-brain oxygen uptake. Similar
results were obtained later with the cerebrospinal fluid displacement
method (Rosenbaum et al. 1942) and with whole-brain cerebral
blood flow using the nitrous oxide technique (Kety et al. 1948).
However, these studies assessed the function of the whole brain and
did not provide information on specific brain regions. The behavioral
and cognitive changes in schizophrenia do not closely resemble the

Research was supported by NIMH Grant MH-40071; a gift from Eldon and
Marjorie Lockhart; and a small grant by Network 3, MacArthur Foundation.
Isotopes were provided by Crocker Laboratory, University of California,
Davis; Dr. Thomas Cahill; Dr. Manuel Lagunas-Solar; Dr. Stanley Mills;
David Manthei; and Katsumi Tomioshi. My collaborators at University of
California, Los Angeles (Kieth Nuechterlein, Robert Asarnow), and Univer-
sity of California, Irvine (Joseph Wu, Richard Haiev, Steven Potkin), fur-
nished patients and ideas in the development of this work.

symptoms seen in states of global brain dysfunction such as hypoglycemia or diabetic acidosis, but, rather, suggest specific regional cortical or subcortical deficits.

Regional metabolic information was first obtained by Ingvar and Franzen (1974), who imaged human cerebral blood flow with xenon-133 in patients with schizophrenia and control subjects. The normal-flow topography was described in the resting subject, with relatively high flows in the frontal lobes and relatively lower flows in temporal and occipital regions. Schizophrenic individuals did not show the hyperfrontal pattern seen in normal individuals. Statistical analyses revealed that neither frontal nor occipital flow rates in themselves showed significant differences between groups and that the ratio between frontal and occipital flows did reach significance (1.10 in normal individuals, 1.04 in younger patients, 0.95 in older patients). Ingvar introduced the term "hypofrontality" to describe this pattern. Use of ratios provides a way to normalize for intersubject variability and has been very useful in localizing regional brain changes in blood flow, EEG, and glucose metabolites.

The first studies with PET in schizophrenic patients focused on the function of the frontal lobes, which had already been shown to be abnormal in schizophrenic patients (Ingvar and Franzen 1974). Furthermore, the important role of the frontal lobes in attention, motivation, and the planning and organizing of behavior could lead, if dysfunctional, to behavioral and cognitive changes similar to those seen in schizophrenic patients. David Ingvar visited the National Institute of Mental Health in Bethesda, Maryland, in 1980; my colleagues and I decided to replicate his 1974 blood-flow studies with fluorodeoxyglucose (FDG) and PET, using a small series of schizophrenic patients who were studied in a resting condition with their eyes closed. This series (Buchsbaum et al. 1982) revealed, like the 1974 data, a diminished frontal/occipital ratio in patients with schizophrenia (1.14 in normal individuals, 1.05 in patients). Similar findings were obtained when studying the patients while they received brief electric shocks to their right forearms (Buchsbaum et al. 1984a) and when studying the patients while they performed the Continuous Performance Test (CPT) (Buchsbaum et al. 1990), as illustrated in Figure 2-1. Since then, several PET studies have investigated function in the frontal regions of schizophrenic patients. In Table 2-1, I provide a summary of these studies. The majority of these reports show relatively low function in the frontal regions of patients with schizophrenia. In Table 2-1, we have compared the results for the different PET studies using the frontal/occipital ratio to facilitate cross-study comparison and to provide evidence for a specific regional pattern rather than global brain metabolic change. We calculated the ratio from the authors' raw data tables or figures when the ratio was not supplied. This summary revealed lower frontal/occipital ratios in 11 of 14 studies. The ratios were significantly lower in schizophrenic patients when compared with normal individuals in five studies (Buchsbaum et al. 1982, 1984a, 1987; Farkas et al. 1984; Wolkin et al. 1988) and either were nonsignificantly lower or could not be tested in six studies (Jernigan et al. 1985; Kishimoto et al. 1987; Kling et al. 1986; Sheppard et al. 1983; Volkow et al. 1987; Wolkin et al. 1985). One study of the 14 reviewed (Szechtman et al. 1988) found significantly higher ratios in patients with schizophrenia, and one review showed a tie (Gur et al. 1987). Cohen et al. (1987) found significantly lower frontal metabolism in schizophrenic patients by analysis of variance (ANOVA) but did not present data from which ratios can be calculated. Early et al. (1987) did not present data in tabular form or in sufficient detail to allow inclusion of the frontal/occipital ratio.

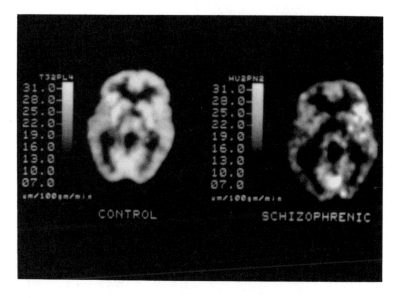

Figure 2-1. PET scan in normal control subject and unmedicated schizophrenic patient. Scale is glucose metabolic rate in micromoles of glucose/100 g brain/minute, adjusted to the maximum and minimum of each slice. Hypofrontal metabolic rate is clearly seen in the frontal region of the patient. Note that the occipital areas are maximum on the patient with schizophrenia but the frontal area is maximum on the normal control subject.

Table 2-1. Comparison of PET studies in schizophrenia

Reference	Frontal/occipital ratio			Frontal/whole-brain ratio			Site in brain	Number of patients	Sensory condition	Medications
	N	S	P	N	S	P				
Buchsbaum et al. 1982	1.14	1.05	<.05[1]	1.12	1.06	<.05	Supraventricular	8	Eyes closed	Off
Buchsbaum et al. 1984	1.08	1.02	<.05[2]	1.14	1.09	<.05	Supraventricular	16	Shocks	Off
Farkas et al. 1984[2]	1.14	1.07	<.05[3]	1.11	1.05	NT	Supraventricular	11	Open room	6[5]
Sheppard et al. 1983[4]	1.1	1.0	NS				OM + 6 cm	12	Eyes closed	6[5]
Jernigan et al. 1985[6]	1.10	1.03	NS	1.03	.98	NS	Midventricular	6	Auditory	Off
Wolkin et al. 1985	1.09	1.04	NS	1.08	1.04	<.05	Midventricular	10	Eyes open	Off
Kling et al. 1986[7]	.79	.74	NS	.97	.92	<.05	"High"	6	Eyes open	On
Weisel et al. 1985[8]				1.16	1.12	NT	Brodmann area 9, 10	13	Eyes closed	Off
Wolkin et al. 1988	1.10	1.04	<.03				Midventricular	13	Eyes open	Off
Volkow et al. 1987	.91	.90	NT[9]	1.01	.98	NT	Frontal lobe	18	Eyes open	On
Szechtman et al. 1988	1.06	1.23	<.01[10]	.97	1.02	NS	Supraventricular	12	Eyes closed	On
Szechtman et al. 1988	1.06	1.31	<.01[11]	.97	1.08	<.05	Supraventricular	5	Eyes closed	Off
Buchsbaum et al. 1987	1.15	1.05	<.01	1.12	1.06	<.05	Midventricular	13	CPT	Off
Gur et al. 1987	1.08	1.08	NS	.77	.72	NT	Frontal lobe	12	Eyes open	Off[12]
Kishimoto et al. 1987	1.09	.92	NT[13]				Brodmann area 10	20	Eyes closed	On

Note. Analysis for right hemisphere, supraventricular slice when available; N = normal; S = schizophrenic; NS = $P > .05$; NT = not tested; OM = orbito-meatal line. Empty cells represent studies that did not provide data to obtain the values for the ratios.

[1] Linear trend analysis of variance (ANOVA).
[2] Right and left combined, calculated from Tables 1–3 of Farkas et al. (1984) article.
[3] Analysis of covariance.
[4] Ratio calculated by authors to only 1 significant figure after decimal.
[5] Six patients not more than 7 days off medication.
[6] Automated analysis.
[7] Frontal/whole slice different by t test.
[8] Occipital data not given in report; frontal areas calculated from Brodmann area 9 and 10 data.
[9] Right frontal rate for schizophrenic patients (35.4) lower than normal subjects (40.0) by t test, $P < .01$.
[10] One-way ANOVA for normal subjects, medicated schizophrenic patients.
[11] Never-medicated schizophrenic patients.
[12] Off medication more than 7 days.
[13] Means calculated by weighted averages from Table 4 of Kishimoto et al. (1987) article.

The ratio of frontal to occipital metabolic rates reflects the function of both the frontal and the occipital lobes, since high occipital values can contribute to hypofrontality. This ratio contrasts the executive functions of the frontal lobe and the sensory processing functions of the occipital lobe. Indeed, in an oversimplified model, the pattern of hypofrontal and hyperoccipital function matches the deficits in planning and organization and the excessive sensory elaboration seen in schizophrenia. Frontal to whole-brain or whole-slice ratios have also been used to investigate regional brain defects in schizophrenic patients. This ratio is less affected by occipital metabolism. Using this ratio, we found six studies that showed significantly lower frontal whole-brain or whole-slice ratios in schizophrenic patients (Buchsbaum et al. 1982, 1984a, 1990; Cohen et al. 1987; Kling et al. 1986; Wolkin et al. 1985) and four others that showed lower ratios that were nonsignificant or not tested statistically (Farkas et al. 1984; Gur et al. 1987; Jernigan et al. 1985; Volkow et al. 1987). Wiesel et al. (1985) found higher ratios for areas 6 and 8 but lower ratios for areas 9 and 10. Szechtman et al. (1988) found significantly higher ratios. Sheppard et al. (1983), Kishimoto et al. (1987), and Early et al. (1987) did not present data making this computation possible.

In our PET studies done in the Genain quadruplets, identical quadruplets concordant for schizophrenia, all four were 1 standard deviation (SD) below normal for the frontal/whole-slice ratio and two were 2 SDs below normal (Buchsbaum et al. 1984b). Though the small size of the sample from this twin study precludes the derivation of any conclusive statements, the consistency of hypofrontality in the four sisters suggests a possible genetic component in hypofrontality and schizophrenia.

A third strategy in analyzing frontal derangements in schizophrenic patients has been to use the absolute values for glucose metabolism (μmol or mg/unit of time) in the frontal lobes. While they do not correct for the wide individual differences in whole-brain metabolic rate, they have the advantage of being entirely independent of other brain areas. Lower cerebral metabolic rates of glucose in schizophrenic patients than in control subjects are reported in 9 of 10 studies (Volkow et al. 1987; Farkas et al. 1984 [our t test, $t = 2.12$, $P < .05$]; Wolkin et al. 1985, Wiesel et al. 1987 [areas 9 and 10 but not areas 6 or 8]; Kling et al. 1986 [high frontal, right posterior inferior frontal]; Cohen et al. 1987, Gur et al. 1987 [3.32 mg/100 g/minute versus 3.98 in normal subjects, our t test, $t = 3.00$, $P < .01$]; Buchsbaum et al. 1987, Kishimoto et al. 1987 [our t test on calculated weighted mean of pixel counts, $t = 2.41$, $P < .05$]). Only Buchsbaum et al. (1984a) found nonsignificantly higher frontal metabolic rates, perhaps because of the use of painful somatosensory stimulation, which may activate the frontal lobes.

Whole-brain or whole-cortical metabolic rates did not differ significantly between normal subjects and schizophrenic patients in six studies, suggesting a specific frontal lobe hypofunction in agreement with the majority of the ratio studies (Buchsbaum et al. 1984a, 1990; Cohen et al. 1987; Farkas et al. 1984; Volkow et al. 1987 [39.7 versus 35.9, our t test, $t = 1.61$, P NS]; Wiesel et al. 1987). However, the data of Gur et al. (1987) did show significant whole-cortical reductions in schizophrenic patients.

Despite the fact that these studies differ widely in uptake conditions, region of interest location and size, medication status of patients, demographic features, and sample size, a modest consistency appears. Variation between studies may also relate to the high levels of Type II statistical errors inherent in these small samples. Nevertheless, the PET data are consistent with the data showing reduced frontal cerebral blood flow (Buchsbaum and Haier 1987), the formulations on the role of the frontal cortex in schizophrenia (Ingvar and Franzen 1974; Levin 1984; Weinberger 1987; Weinberger et al. 1988), and the heterogeneity of schizophrenic diathesis (Buchsbaum and Rieder 1979).

MAGNITUDE OF RELATIVE HYPOFRONTALITY

While the size of the difference between schizophrenic patients and normal subjects may appear small (1.06 versus 1.13 in the original Ingvar and Franzen study in 1974), it must be assessed in terms of group-difference contrasts. The size of the effect can be assessed by examining the diminution of the anteroposterior gradient in patients as a percentage of normal, the relative relationship to one SD in normal subjects, and the sensitivity and specificity in contrast to other biological marker studies. The modest effect size must also be considered in the context of the biological heterogeneity of patients with schizophrenia (Buchsbaum and Haier 1983; Buchsbaum and Rieder 1979).

Percentage Loss

Patients with schizophrenia show a loss of about two-thirds of the normal anteroposterior gradient. The normal front-to-back gradient (frontal lobe sector/occipital lobe sector) is 11% (1.15–1.04, right side, levels combined, Buchsbaum et al. 1990) but only 3% (1.10–1.07) in schizophrenic patients (a 27% reduction from normal). Similar contrasts are seen in examining metabolic rate, where normal subjects show a gradient of 2.2 µM/100 g/minute (22.1 frontal lobe—19.9 occipital lobe, right side, levels combined, Buchsbaum et al. 1990), but schizophrenic patients show a gradient of 0.5 (18.5–18.0) (a 23% reduction from normal). The change in gradient from 2.2 to 0.5 is 1.7 μM/100 g per minute, which is 8% of the normal frontal metabolic rate. It is interesting to compare the magnitude of this change with the magnitude of the brain change observed when using brain stimulation paradigms. For example, the cortical metabolic rate change with painful electric shock was 1.68 μM, a change of 6% (Buchsbaum et al. 1983), and the difference between eyes closed and eyes open was 10% (Phelps et al. 1981).

Effect Size

The effect size for the right anterior/posterior ratio in standard units is 1.10 (1.18 in normal subjects, 1.07 in patients; SD = 0.10). This is in the same range as the other blood-flow and PET studies reviewed elsewhere (Buchsbaum and Haier 1987) and in the effect size range expected by statisticians for psychiatric studies (Bartko et al. 1988).

Sensitivity and Specificity of Hypofrontality

We examined this using the frontal/occipital ratio of 1.05 as a cutoff score, a level found to be a useful criterion in our 1982 and 1984 NIMH studies (Figure 2-2). For the infraventricular slice, we identified 7 of 13 schizophrenic patients, but only 1 of 17 normal patients, as hypofrontal (Figure 2-2). This yields a sensitivity of 53% and a specificity of 94% (Kalter et al. 1983). The sensitivity parallels the

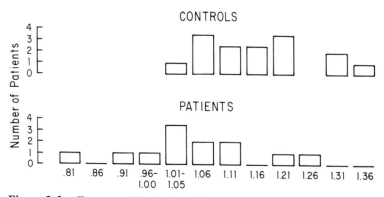

Figure 2-2. Frequency distribution of the right frontal/right occipital ratio in 17 normal subjects and 13 off-medication patients with schizophrenia. Criterion of less than or equal to 1.05 is used to separate groups, a criterion derived from earlier studies (Buchsbaum et al. 1984a).

finding that poor CPT results characterize about half of schizophrenic inpatients (Orzack and Kornetsky 1966; Walker and Shaye 1982). The CPT is a visual vigilance task that involves monitoring a series of briefly presented stimuli (usually numbers or letters) that appear one at a time at a rapid serial rate and signaling by a button press each time a predesignated target stimulus is presented. The CPT shows high reliability on repeat testing and is, therefore, suitable for studies of trait features (Cornblatt et al. 1988). For our 1984 data (electric shock stimulation during study), we found 11 of 16 schizophrenic patients to be hypofrontal, but only 7 of 19 of the control subjects; this is a sensitivity of 68% and a specificity of 63%. The use of the CPT during the PET study (Buchsbaum et al. 1990) appeared to enhance the specificity without changing sensitivity. The enhancement of specificity probably reflects the value of using a task that is performed abnormally by schizophrenic patients. We also applied the 1.05 criterion to the data of Wolkin et al. (1985). This identified 6 of 10 schizophrenic patients but only 1 of 8 normal subjects, a sensitivity of 60% and a specificity of 88%. The only published blood-flow distributions of hypofrontality indices are those of Weinberger et al. (1988). If we apply the same 1.05 cutoff point, then 7 of 16 schizophrenic patients, but only 2 of 25 control subjects, are hypofrontal. This is a sensitivity of 44% and a specificity of 92%. These figures are very similar to ours and in the range of those reported for other biological tests in psychiatry (see review by Buchsbaum and Haier 1983).

HEMISPHERIC LATERALITY

In our study using the CPT (Buchsbaum et al. 1990), normal subjects showed a higher right versus left metabolic rate for the whole-hemisphere cortical surface, and this difference was larger during active execution of the CPT task than during passive stimulus viewing. In contrast, patients with schizophrenia failed to show the asymmetry. The higher metabolic activity in the right hemisphere of normal subjects is located on average in the superior and middle temporal gyrus and inferior anterior parietal lobe (Brodmann's areas 40, 41, 42, 22, 37, 27, and part of 39).

Our observation of a slightly higher metabolic rate in the cortex of the right hemisphere is consistent with the majority of PET studies of normal subjects tested under resting conditions or when using nonlateralized sensory activation. Eight studies showed the right hemisphere to be greater than the left, three with statistical confirmation (Buchsbaum et al. 1983; Perlmutter et al. 1987; Wiesel et al. 1985) and five without (de Leon et al. 1984; Emrich et al. 1984; Gur et al. 1987; Jernigan et al. 1985; Wiesel et al. 1987). Six studies showed the left hemisphere to be greater than the right, only one with statistical confirmation (Baxter et al. 1985) and five without (Baxter et al. 1987; Kling et al. 1986; Rumsey et al. 1985; Volkow et al. 1987; Wolkin et al. 1985). Two studies showed hemispheres equal or varying in right or left predominance (Szechtman et al. 1988; Wolkin et al. 1988).

Patients with schizophrenia in PET studies who were compared with control subjects who were more right than left active (or with equal activity in right and left hemispheres) were relatively less right-activated than control subjects in five studies (Buchsbaum et al. 1983, 1988; Jernigan et al. 1985; Wiesel et al. 1987; Wolkin et al. 1988) and equally right-activated in two (Gur et al. 1987; Wiesel et al. 1985). However, patients in studies who were compared with control subjects who were more left-activated than right (all with eyes open) showed relatively greater right-activation (Kling et al. 1986 for low frontal region; Volkow et al. 1987; Wolkin et al. 1985). Wik et al. (1989) found right greater than left for control subjects and non-medicated patients statistically confirmed for Brodmann area 6 alone. These shifts are small and not uniformly evaluated statistically in these reports. However, they suggest that schizophrenic patients may have different lateralization patterns than control subjects and that having them do a specific task during uptake may be crucial for exploring hemispheric contrasts. It is also interesting that the report of Kishimoto et al. (1987) showed a subgroup of patients with distinctly reduced right parietal metabolic rates.

While the perceptually degraded nature of the stimuli presented during the CPT used in our study (Buchsbaum et al. 1987) may be a contributor to the greater right hemisphere activation (Hellige 1982; Moscovitch 1979; Sergent 1983), the demand for ongoing vigilance that characterizes the CPT may also be important. The right hemisphere may have a larger role in regulating overall attentional tone than the left hemisphere (Mesulam 1985). Last, it is possible that vigilance tasks may not be entirely dissimilar to the demand for vigilance that an unfamiliar environment such as the PET laboratory requires. This similarity could explain the success in demonstrating hypofrontality among the many functional imaging studies that tested subjects at rest.

RELATIVE FRONTAL LOBE HYPOFUNCTION AND TASK

In general, these studies have tended to show that patients with schizophrenia had lower frontal/occipital ratios than normal individuals, although it was not confirmed to a statistically significant extent in all of the other studies. However, both PET and blood-flow studies have been variable in the extent to which the hypofrontal differences are manifest. In some cases, while schizophrenic patients had lower ratios, these ratios were still above 1.00, leading to the term "relative hypofrontality."

Important sources of variation that have been suggested are the psychological state and the environmental influences during the PET study. Given the sensitivity of both cerebral blood flow and FDG to external stimulation, uncontrolled sensory and perceptual input during the PET study might well influence the pattern of cerebral brain metabolism, and this influence may be different in schizophrenic patients than in normal individuals.

To control this source of variation, we selected somatosensory stimulation for our second PET study (Buchsbaum et al. 1984a). Pain stimulation had been reported to increase frontal lobe blood flow in humans (Ingvar et al. 1976) and animals (Tsubokawa et al. 1981) and to reveal diminished pain sensitivity and diminished evoked potential amplitude in patients with schizophrenia (Buchsbaum et al. 1986; Davis et al. 1979a, 1979b). Pain stimulation during FDG uptake continued to reveal statistically significant differences in relative frontal/occipital metabolic rate. However, it did not alter frontal/occipital ratios from the resting state in normal subjects (Buchsbaum et al. 1983) at the supraventricular level of the cortex (Brodmann areas 10, 11, 46, and part of 45), where we had observed our patient-normal differences. Thus, while perhaps useful for controlling sensory condition and thus reducing variance, the shock condition did not specifically activate the brain regions targeted for study (although the "rest" condition might not be optimal for comparison).

For our third study (Buchsbaum et al. 1990), we selected the CPT because this task has shown particular sensitivity to schizophrenic performance deficit.

Patients with schizophrenia show a greater percentage of correct target detections on the CPT than do normal subjects, chronic alcoholic patients (see review in Buchsbaum et al. 1990), or patients with schizoaffective disorder or major affective disorders (Cornblatt et al. 1989; Walker 1981). The CPT deficit appears in about half of schizophrenic patients (Orzack and Kornetsky 1966; Walker and Shaye 1982). Patients with CPT deficit are more likely to have a family history of schizophrenia (Walker and Shaye 1982) or serious mental illness (Orzack and Kornetsky 1971) than are schizophrenic patients who are good CPT performers. Patients at risk for schizophrenia also show poor CPT performance (Erlenmeyer-Kimling and Cornblatt

1978; Rutschmann et al. 1977). The relative sensitivity of the CPT to attentional impairment among children at heightened risk for schizophrenia is also suggested by the finding that the CPT score on perceptual sensitivity (d') produced significant differences between children of schizophrenic mothers and representative normal children, whereas measures from cross-modal reaction time and incidental learning tasks did not (Nuechterlein et al. 1982).

Deficits in target detection rate and false-alarm rate have been demonstrated in both stable postpsychotic schizophrenic outpatients on antipsychotic medication (Asarnow and MacCrimmon 1978) and schizophrenic patients off medication tested during remission while functioning at their premorbid level (Wohlberg and Kornetsky 1973). Thus, cross-sectional studies at premorbid, psychotic, and postpsychotic points suggest that some persons prone to schizophrenia might manifest CPT deficits throughout their life course.

PET studies that have evaluated frontal lobe function in schizophrenic patients tested in resting and in performing conditions have shown larger differences from normal individuals when patients were tested during task conditions. Our own current data (Buchsbaum et al. 1990) show the whole frontal lobe both relatively and absolutely lower in schizophrenic patients tested during the degraded-stimulus CPT, while scans from schizophrenic patients tested during resting (Buchsbaum et al. 1982) showed significance only on the ratio measure obtained at the supraventricular level. In another vigilance study, an auditory discrimination task not dissimilar to the visual CPT was used during FDG uptake in normal subjects and patients with schizophrenia (Cohen et al. 1987). A marked decrease in metabolic rates in the prefrontal cortex of schizophrenic patients was found, even among those patients with performance in the normal range. A correlation between metabolic rate in middle prefrontal cortex and accuracy of performance was found in normal subjects. Cerebral blood flow during the Wisconsin Card Sort Test showed stronger evidence of hypofrontality than during rest (Weinberger et al. 1986), although resting schizophrenic patients were significantly hypofrontal as well (confirmed by ANOVA; ratios 1.12 in normal subjects and 1.07 in schizophrenic patients). However, Volkow et al. (1987) used an eye tracking task and found only slightly larger frontal/whole-brain ratio differences during the task (normal subjects = 1.00, schizophrenic patients = 0.97) than during baseline (normal subjects = 1.01, schizophrenic patients = 0.98), and this difference was not statistically contrasted. In reviewing this task work it should be emphasized that so far cerebral blood-flow studies have used whole frontal lobe measures from several flow probes and most PET studies have similarly not exploited their available resolution. Studies of frontal lobe tasks such as the Wisconsin Card Sort Test have found that lesions of the medial, dorsolateral, and orbital regions show different kinds of deficits, and hemisphere of lesion is also important (e.g., Drewe 1974). Drewe notes that it is the medial frontal area and not the dorsolateral convexity that is a critical area for some aspects of the test. Last, it should be noted that the use of a task that does not specifically activate the frontal lobe could reduce or eliminate the finding of hypofrontality but emphasize other brain-region deficits.

EFFECTS OF NEUROLEPTICS ON FRONTAL LOBE METABOLISM

Consistent with the distribution of dopamine receptors in the brain, most studies of cerebral metabolism have shown greater effects of dopaminergic drugs on the basal ganglia than on the frontal lobe. In animal studies, manipulation of the dopaminergic system with 6-hydroxydopamine injections produced changes in subcortical structures but not in the frontal lobes (Kozlowski and Marshall 1980), a finding similar to later studies (Wooten and Collins 1981). We found a significant increase in metabolic rate in the putamen but no statistically significant change in the anteroposterior ratio in eight schizophrenic patients scanned both on and off neuroleptics (1.06 on medication, 1.04 off medication, $t = 0.34$, P NS, Buchsbaum et al. 1987). No cortical area showed a statistically significant increase, although a trend ($P < .10$) appeared toward increased metabolic rates. (An earlier study using one additional patient who was tested in a different condition was omitted from this analysis; this report [DeLisi et al. 1985] showed a small increase in cortical metabolism.) Further, significant correlations were found between basal ganglia metabolic change with medication and Brief Psychiatric Rating Scale (Overall and Gorham 1962) improvement. Cohen et al. (1988) found increases in basal ganglia metabolic rate with neuroleptics as we did, with little effect in the frontal lobes. Interestingly, neuroleptic effects appeared primarily in areas of the brain not correlated with performance on the CPT. Increased metabolism in the lentiform nucleus with the antipsychotic sulpiride, a drug with several similarities to clozapine, was also found by Wik et al. (1989). This effect was greatest in the right, just as we had observed (Buchsbaum et al. 1987). Gur et al. (1987) found no effect of neuroleptics on the frontal lobe but did not show basal ganglia effects either (Gur et al. 1987; Resnick et al. 1988). The frontal lobe was one of the few areas that failed to show a significant neuroleptic effect in the study by Wolkin et al. (1985), but the increase in occipital metabolic rate produced a statistically significant decrease in the hypofrontality ratio. Wiesel et al. (1985) and Wik et al. (1989) also reported no significant effect of sulpiride treatment on the frontal lobe. Volkow et al. (1986) found no effects of neuroleptics anywhere in the brain but studied only four patients (Type II error estimated at 91%). However, it should be noted that no study administered a fixed dose of neuroleptics for a fixed interval in a placebo-controlled random assignment trial; all followed drug-withdrawn patients subsequently treated, confounding order and drug treatment. Analysis of data from a controlled design from patients performing a task sensitive to the effects of neuroleptics is clearly needed to resolve this issue.

CONCLUSION

Like the findings of increased ventricular ratio, the finding of reduced frontal lobe function in schizophrenia is now becoming widely replicated. However, it is similarly variable in extent and not fully specific in anatomical locale, and its pathophysiology is not fully understood. The weak statistical nature of the finding and its low sensitivity may reflect the underlying heterogeneity of the biology of schizophrenia, the variability of functional states over time, measurement errors inherent in scanning, and glucose quantification. Further, phenocopies of genetic schizophrenia such as head injury, anoxic damage, and even viral infection may also be associated with reduced frontal lobe function. These possibilities may be further evaluated by more specific anatomical localization within the frontal lobe. With PET resolution in the current 5- to 10-mm range, a far more detailed picture of the finding can be constructed. This, combined with studies of drug response, will help to reveal aspects of the pathophysiology of hypofrontality.

REFERENCES

Asarnow RF, MacCrimmon DJ: Residual performance deficit in clinically remitted schizophrenics: a marker of schizophrenia. J Abnorm Psychol 87:597–608, 1978

Bartko JJ, Pulver AE, Carpenter WT Jr: The power of analysis: statistical perspectives, part 2. Psychiatry Res 23:301–310, 1988

Baxter LR, Phelps ME, Mazziotta JC, et al: Cerebral metabolic rates for glucose in mood disorders (studies with positron emission tomography and fluorodeoxyglucose F-18). Arch Gen Psychiatry 42:441–447, 1985

Baxter LR, Mazziotta JC, Phelps ME, et al: Cerebral glucose metabolic rates in normal human females versus normal males. Psychiatry Res 21:237–245, 1987

Buchsbaum MS, Haier RJ: Psychopathology: biological approaches. Ann Rev Psychol 34:401–430, 1983

Buchsbaum MS, Haier RJ: Functional and anatomical brain imaging: impact on schizophrenia research. Schizophr Bull 13:115–132, 1987

Buchsbaum MS, Rieder RO: Biologic heterogeneity and psychiatric research: platelet MAO as a case study. Arch Gen Psychiatry 36:1163–1169, 1979

Buchsbaum MS, Ingvar DH, Kessler R, et al: Cerebral glucography with positron emission tomography. Arch Gen Psychiatry 39:251–259, 1982

Buchsbaum MS, Holcomb HH, Johnson J, et al: Cerebral metabolic consequences of electrical cutaneous stimulation in normal individuals. Human Neurobiology 2:35–38, 1983

Buchsbaum MS, DeLisi LE, Holcomb HH, et al: Anteroposterior gradients in cerebral glucose use in schizophrenia and affective disorders. Arch Gen Psychiatry 41:1159–1166, 1984a

Buchsbaum MS, Mirsky AF, DeLisi LE, et al: The Genain quadruplets: electrophysiological, positron emission and X-ray tomographic studies. Psychiatry Res 13:95–108, 1984b

Buchsbaum MS, Awsare SV, Holcomb HH, et al: Topographic differences between normals and schizophrenics: the N120 evoked potential component. Neuropsychobiology 15:1–6, 1986

Buchsbaum MS, Wu JC, DeLisi LE, et al: Positron emission tomography studies of basal ganglia and somatosensory cortex neuroleptic drug effects: differences between normal controls and schizophrenic patients. Biol Psychiatry 22:479–494, 1987

Buchsbaum MS, Nuechterlein KH, Haier RJ, et al: Glucose metabolic rate in normals and schizophrenics during the continuous performance test assessed by positron emission tomography. Br J Psychiatry 156:216–227, 1990

Cohen RM, Semple WE, Gross M, et al: Dysfunction in a prefrontal substrate of sustained attention in schizophrenia. Life Sci 40:2031–2039, 1987

Cohen RM, Semple WE, Gross M, et al: The effect of neuroleptics on dysfunction in a prefrontal substrate of sustained attention in schizophrenia. Life Sci 43:1141–1150, 1988

Cornblatt BA, Risch NJ, Faris G, et al: The Continuous Performance Test, Identical Pairs version (CPT-IP): new findings about sustained attention in normal families. Psychiatry Res 26:223–238, 1988

Cornblatt BA, Lenzenweger MF, Erlenmeyer-Kimling L: The Continuous Performance Test, Identical Pairs Version (CPT-IP), II: contrasting attentional profiles in schizophrenic and depressed patients. Psychiatry Res 29:65–86, 1989

Davis GC, Buchsbaum MS, Bunney WE Jr: Research in endorphins and schizophrenia. Schizophr Bull 5:244–250, 1979a

Davis GC, Buchsbaum MS, van Kammen DP, et al: Analgesia to pain stimuli in schizophrenics and its reversal by naltrexone. Psychiatry Res 1:61–69, 1979b

De Leon MJ, George AE, Ferris SH, et al: Positron emission tomography and computed tomography assessments of the aging human brain. J Comput Assist Tomogr 8:88–94, 1984

DeLisi LE, Holcomb HH, Cohen RM, et al: Positron emission tomography in schizophrenic patients with and without neuroleptic medication. J Cereb Blood Flow Metab 5:201–206, 1985

Drewe EA: The effect of type and area of brain lesion on Wisconsin Card Sorting Test performance. Cortex 10:159, 1974

Early TS, Reiman EM, Raichle ME, et al: Left globus pallidus abnormality in never-medicated patients with schizophrenia. Proc Natl Acad Sci USA 84:561–563, 1987

Emrich HM, Pahl JJ, Herholz K, et al: PET investigation in anorexia nervosa: normal glucose metabolism during pseudoatrophy of the brain, in The Psychobiology of Anorexia Nervosa. Edited by Pirke KM, Ploog D. Berlin-Heidelberg, Springer-Verlag, 1984, pp 172–178

Erlenmeyer-Kimling L, Cornblatt B: Attentional measures in a study of children at high risk for schizophrenia. J Psychiatr Res 14:93–98, 1978

Farkas T, Wolf AP, Jaeger J, et al: Regional brain glucose metabolism in chronic schizophrenia: a positron emission transaxial tomographic study. Arch Gen Psychiatry 41:293–300, 1984

Gur RE, Resnick SM, Alavi A, et al: Regional brain function in schizophrenia: positron emission tomography study. Arch Gen Psychiatry 44:119–125, 1987

Hellige JB: Visual laterality and hemisphere specialization: methodological and theoretical considerations, in Conditioning, Cognition, and Methodology: Contemporary Issues in Experimental Psychology. Hillsdale, NJ, Lawrence Erlbaum, 1982

Himwich HD, Bowman KM, Wortis J, et al: Biochemical changes occurring in the cerebral blood during the insulin treatment of schizophrenia. J Nerv Ment Dis 89:273–293, 1939

Ingvar DH, Franzen G: Abnormalities of cerebral blood flow distribution in patients with chronic schizophrenia. Acta Psychiatr Scand 50:425–462, 1974

Ingvar DH, Rosen I, Eriksson M, et al: Activation patterns induced in the dominant hemisphere by skin stimulation, in Sensory Functions of the Skin. Edited by Zotterman Y. London, Pergamon, 1976, pp 549–559

Jernigan TL, Sargent T III, Pfefferbaum A, et al: 18-Fluorodeoxyglucose PET in schizophrenia. Psychiatry Res 16:317–330, 1985

Kalter N, Feinberg M, Carroll BJ: Inferential statistical methods for strengthening the interpretation of laboratory test results. Psychiatry Res 10:207–216, 1983

Kety SS, Woodford RB, Harmel MH, et al: Cerebral blood flow and metabolism in schizophrenia: the effects of barbiturate semi-narcosis, insulin, coma and electroshock. Am J Psychiatry 104:765–770, 1947–48

Kishimoto H, Kuwahara H, Ohno S, et al: Three subtypes of chronic schizophrenia identified using ^{11}C-glucose positron emission tomography. Psychiatry Res 21:285–292, 1987

Kling AS, Metter EJ, Riege WH, et al: Comparison of PET measurement of local brain glucose metabolism and CAT measurement of brain atrophy in chronic schizophrenia and depression. Am J Psychiatry 143:175–180, 1986

Kozlowski MR, Marshall JF: Plasticity of [^{14}C]2-deoxy-D-glucose incorporation into neostriatum and related structures in response to dopamine neuron damage and apomorphine replacement. Brain Res 197:167–183, 1980

Levin S: Frontal lobe dysfunctions in schizophrenia, I: eye movement impairments. J Psychiatr Res 18:27–55, 1984

Mesulam M-M: Attention, confusional states, and neglect, in Principles of Behavioral Neurology. Edited by Mesulam M-M. Philadelphia, PA, FA Davis, 1985

Moscovitch M: Information processing in the cerebral hemispheres, in Handbook of Behavioral Neurobiology, Vol 2: Neuropsychology. Edited by Gazzaniga MS. New York, Plenum, 1979

Nuechterlein KH: Signal detection in vigilance tasks and behavioral attributes among offspring of schizophrenic mothers and among hyperactive children. J Abnorm Psychol 92:4–28, 1983

Nuechterlein KH, Phipps-Yonas S, Driscoll RM, et al: The role of different components of attention in children vulnerable to schizophrenia, in

Preventive Intervention in Schizophrenia: Are We Ready? Edited by Goldstein MJ. Washington, DC, U.S. Government Printing Office, 1982

Orzack M, Kornetsky C: Attention dysfunction in chronic schizophrenia. Arch Gen Psychiatry 14:323–326, 1966

Orzack M, Kornetsky C: Environmental and familial predictors of attention behavior in chronic schizophrenics. J Psychiatr Res 9:21–29, 1971

Overall JE, Gorham DR: The Brief Psychiatric Rating Scale. Psychol Rep 10:799–812, 1962

Perlmutter JS, Powers WJ, Herscovitch P, et al: Regional asymmetries of cerebral blood flow, blood volume, and oxygen utilization and extraction in normal subjects. J Cereb Blood Flow Metab 7:64–67, 1987

Phelps ME, Mazziotta JC, Kuhl DE, et al: Tomographic mapping of human cerebral metabolism: visual stimulation and deprivation. Neurology 31:517–529, 1981

Resnick SM, Gur RE, Alavi A, et al: Positron emission tomography and subcortical glucose metabolism in schizophrenia. Psychiatry Res 24:1–11, 1988

Rosenbaum M, Roseman E, Airing CD, et al: Intracranial blood flow in dementia paralytica, cerebral atrophy and schizophrenia. Archives of Neurology and Psychiatry 47:793–799, 1942

Rumsey JM, Duara R, Grady C, et al: Brain metabolism in autism. Arch Gen Psychiatry 42:448–455, 1985

Rutschmann J, Cornblatt G, Erlenmeyer-Kimling L: Sustained attention in children at risk for schizophrenia. Arch Gen Psychiatry 34:571–575, 1977

Sergent J: Role of the input in visual hemispheric asymmetries. Psychol Bull 93:481–512, 1983

Sheppard G, Gruzelier J, Manchanda R, et al: Positron emission tomographic scanning in predominantly never-treated acute schizophrenic patients. Lancet 2:1448–1452, 1983

Szechtman HJ, Nahmias C, Garnett ES, et al: Effect of neuroleptics on altered cerebral glucose metabolism in schizophrenia. Arch Gen Psychiatry 45:523–532, 1988

Tsubokawa T, Katayama Y, Ueno Y, et al: Evidence for involvement of the frontal cortex in pain-related cerebral events in cats: increase in local cerebral blood flow by noxious stimuli. Brain Res 217:179–185, 1981

Volkow ND, Brodie JD, Wolf AP, et al: Brain metabolism in patients with schizophrenia before and after acute neuroleptic administration. J Neurol Neurosurg Psychiatry 49:1190–1202, 1986

Volkow ND, Wolf AP, van Gelder P, et al: Phenomenological correlates of metabolic activity in 18 patients with chronic schizophrenia. Am J Psychiatry 144:151–158, 1987

Walker E: Attentional and neuromotor functions of schizophrenics, schizoaffectives, and patients with other affective disorders. Arch Gen Psychiatry 38:1355–1358, 1981

Walker E, Shaye J: Familial schizophrenia: a predictor of neuromotor and attentional abnormalities in schizophrenia. Arch Gen Psychiatry 39:1153–1156, 1982

Weinberger DR: Implications of normal brain development for the pathogenesis of schizophrenia. Arch Gen Psychiatry 44:660–669, 1987

Weinberger DR, Berman KF, Zec RF: Physiological dysfunction of dorsolateral prefrontal cortex in schizophrenia, I: regional cerebral blood flow evidence. Arch Gen Psychiatry 43:114–124, 1986

Weinberger DR, Berman KF, Illowsky BP: Physiological dysfunction of dorsolateral prefrontal cortex in schizophrenia. Arch Gen Psychiatry 45:609–615, 1988

Wiesel F-A, Blomqvist G, Greitz T, et al: Proceedings of the 4th World Congress of Biological Psychiatry. New York, Elsevier Science, 1985

Wiesel FA, Wik G, Blomquist SG, et al: Regional brain glucose metabolism in drug free schizophrenic patients and clinical correlates. Acta Psychiatr Scand 76:628–641, 1987

Wik G, Wiesel FA, Sjogren I, et al: Effects of sulpiride and chlorpromazine on regional cerebral glucose metabolism in schizophrenic patients as determined by positron emission tomography. Psychopharmacology 97:309–318, 1989

Wohlberg GW, Kornetsky C: Sustained attention in remitted schizophrenics. Arch Gen Psychiatry 28:533–537, 1973

Wolkin A, Jaeger J, Brodie JD, et al: Persistence of cerebral metabolic abnormalities in chronic schizophrenia as determined by positron emission tomography. Am J Psychiatry 142:564–571, 1985

Wolkin A, Angrist B, Wolf A, et al: Low frontal glucose utilization in chronic schizophrenia: a replication study. Am J Psychiatry 145:251–253, 1988

Wooten GF, Collins RC: Metabolic effects of unilateral lesion of the substantia nigra. J Neurobiol 1:285–291, 1981

Wortis J, Bowman KM, Goldfarb W: Human brain metabolism: normal values and values in certain clinical states. Am J Psychiatry 97:552–565, 1940–41

Chapter 3

Laterality in Schizophrenia: Positron-Emission Tomography Studies

Raquel E. Gur, M.D., Ph.D.,
and Ruben C. Gur, Ph.D.

The application of neuroimaging methods to the study of brain function in schizophrenia has enabled examination of brain regions related to the disorder. A number of brain dimensions have been studied, principally the anterior-posterior (the "hypofrontality hypothesis"), subcortical-cortical, and laterality. In this chapter, we review positron-emission tomography (PET) studies that have tested the hypothesis of lateralized abnormality of brain activity in schizophrenia.

Lateralized abnormalities have been investigated with other neuropsychological and psychophysiological research methods (Gur 1983). This literature suggests that in schizophrenia there is a disturbance in the hemispheric balance of brain function, implicating greater involvement of the left hemisphere.

The focus on laterality is partly related to the vast literature on lateralization of brain function in normal and pathological states. Through careful documentation of neurobehavioral deficits following focal brain lesions, hemispheric functioning has been defined, and variability in relation to handedness and gender was established. This research has yielded several methods for neurobehavioral measurement that permit inferences on hemispheric functioning. These methods range from measures of motoric functions to experimental manipulations. The latter include the tachistoscopic technique for hemifield stimulation (Kimura and Milner 1967), the dichotic listening paradigm for auditory studies of lateralized functioning, and the conjugate lateral eye movement paradigm. These methods were applied to neurologic populations with lateralized disturbance and normal subjects, and lateralized performance indices can be derived for inferring hemispheric capacity and activity (Gur and Reivich

1980). When schizophrenia was examined with these techniques, disturbed laterality was suggested (Flor-Henry et al. 1983). Gur (1978) proposed, on the basis of these techniques, that schizophrenia is associated with left hemispheric dysfunction and an activation imbalance reflecting left hemispheric overactivation.

PET provides an opportunity to evaluate the physiological substrates of lateralized brain function. Unfortunately, not all PET studies have systematically looked at this dimension, and some studies have not used the appropriate procedures for testing the laterality hypothesis. We briefly summarize studies that did address laterality and present our own series of studies designed to test the laterality hypothesis.

GLUCOSE METABOLISM

The majority of PET studies in schizophrenia to date have measured glucose metabolism using the ^{18}F-labeled fluorodeoxyglucose ([^{18}F]FDG) or ^{11}C-labeled deoxyglucose techniques. Buchsbaum et al. (1982) measured brain glucose metabolism in eight unmedicated patients with schizophrenia and six normal control subjects. Subjects were studied with their eyes closed. Patients showed a relative decreased uptake in the left compared with the right cortex. They also had higher activity in the left temporal lobe and lower metabolism in the left basal ganglia. In a subsequent study, with the same radiotracer, Buchsbaum et al. (1984) compared 16 unmedicated patients with schizophrenia with 11 depressed patients and 19 control subjects. During uptake, the subjects' eyes were closed and they received a series of unpleasant electrical stimuli to the right forearm. Data analysis for all slices combined showed no overall group differences or interactions in comparing the three groups using analysis of variance (ANOVA) (Group × Slice Level × Hemisphere × Anterior-Posterior). However, when the midanterior segments were examined, normal control subjects showed a significant asymmetry for the two top slices, with the left higher than the right. By contrast, patients with schizophrenia had the reverse asymmetry on these slices and the difference in asymmetry between patients and control subjects was statistically significant. It is possible that the lack of overall asymmetry was produced by opposite effects in some lower slices. This has not been examined, and the legitimacy of such an analysis can be questioned in view of the lack of a significant four-way interaction. However, it should be kept in mind that the four-way ANOVA included patients with depression that could have masked a significant difference between the patients with schizophrenia and normal control subjects.

In a sample of nine chronic patients studied off and on medications, DeLisi et al. (1985) noted that an increase in cerebral glucose metabolism with treatment was particularly pronounced in the left temporal lobe. A more recent publication examined laterality in greater detail using several approaches to the data analysis. A sample of 21 patients off neuroleptics was compared with 19 control subjects with eyes closed, using a somatosensory stimulation to the right forearm paradigm (DeLisi et al. 1989). Patients had significantly higher glucose metabolism in the temporal lobes, left greater than right. This asymmetry was not observed in normal subjects.

A sample of 18 patients on neuroleptics was compared with 12 control subjects by Volkow et al. (1986a). Subjects were studied with ears plugged and while performing an eye tracking task during the first 30 minutes of uptake. Factor analysis of the metabolic activity suggested four factors, one of which was laterality. This factor did not differ between groups, failing to support the left hemisphere hypothesis. However, in a subsequent study (Volkow et al. 1987), 18 male patients with schizophrenia were compared with 12 male control subjects during resting and the visual task activation paradigm. Results related to hemispheric functioning suggested that patients with predominantly negative symptoms had significantly lower right frontal activity during the task condition. The correlations between glucose metabolism and the dimension of positive and negative symptoms were higher for left hemispheric cortical regions than for homotopic regions in the right hemisphere. In the same laboratory, PET was used to evaluate pharmacologic intervention in four males with schizophrenia, three neuroleptic naive and one treated for 3 months a year earlier. Following a baseline study, thiothixene was injected and the study was repeated. After drug administration, metabolic activity increased in the right basal ganglia only (Volkow et al. 1986b).

Cleghorn et al. (1989) studied a sample of 8 neuroleptic-naive patients and 10 control subjects. No laterality effects were found, but correlations between left frontal and right parietal activity were significant for patients only. In a follow-up of a larger sample with 5 patients treated for 1 year and 12 treated for 4–14 years, no laterality differences emerged (Szechtman et al. 1988).

Wiesel et al. (1987) examined 20 patients off medications and 10 control subjects with eyes closed and ears occluded at uptake. Hemispheric asymmetries were found in the temporal and basal frontal cortices, with lower metabolism on the left in patients relative to control subjects. Examination of diagnostic subgroups revealed higher metabolism in the left amygdala of paranoid patients and in the right amygdala of hebephrenics. The laterality effect was related to duration of treatment.

The effects of sulpiride and chlorpromazine on regional glucose metabolism were evaluated by Wik et al. (1989) in 17 patients. Sulpiride increased metabolic activity in the right lentiform nucleus.

CEREBRAL BLOOD FLOW AND OXYGEN METABOLISM

Two studies have applied PET methodology to the measurement of local cerebral blood flow (CBF) and oxygen metabolism. Sheppard et al. (1983) studied 12 patients and 12 normal control subjects with eyes closed. Patients showed relatively higher left hemispheric oxygen metabolism, supporting the hypothesis of left hemispheric overactivation. Early et al. (1987) reported increased CBF in the left globus pallidus in a sample of 5 neuroleptic-naive patients compared with 10 normal control subjects.

NEURORECEPTOR STUDIES

Farde et al. (1987) evaluated D_2 receptor function using ^{11}C-labeled raclopride in 15 neuroleptic-naive patients and 14 normal control subjects. They reported that in 4 patients and none of the control subjects, D_2 receptor density was 10–30% higher in the left putamen relative to the right.

Several observations can be made on these studies. Most important, the application of the complex PET methodology to small heterogeneous samples under differing study conditions and methods of quantitation and statistical analysis is unlikely to yield robust and systematic data essential for hypothesis testing. This does not reflect poor scientific skills of investigators but rather the preliminary stage of development of the PET technology, particularly its application to neuropsychiatric disorders. The heterogeneity of schizophrenia, manifested in such important clinical variables as symptom type, chronicity, and medication status, requires a particularly cautious approach and a detailed examination of clinical data.

STIMULATION CONDITION IN PET STUDIES

Another issue that merits special attention in physiologic neuroimaging studies is the subject's stimulation condition. Unlike anatomic measures, neurophysiologic parameters are sensitive to environmental effects and can be influenced by cognitive activity (Gur et al. 1982) and emotional or anxiety states (Gur et al. 1988). This has to be considered in constructing PET studies. For example, with other methods it was found that abnormalities were evident not in resting states but in the pattern of response to cognitive activation (Gur et al. 1983, 1985; Weinberger et al. 1986). The "optimal" resting condition is also unclear. Some studies have used eyes open and others have measured "resting" conditions with eyes closed and ears plugged. Yet other studies have deliberately employed sensory stimulation, including electric shocks, because of a methodologic concern that a true unstimulated state is too poorly defined and, hence, useless for systematic examination. In our opinion, sensory deprivation and sensory stimulation have potentially powerful effects on regional brain activity. Unless these effects are isolated, they will confound attempts to examine the laterality hypothesis.

With these limitations in mind, it is noteworthy that the majority of studies with a sufficient sample size that have examined laterality did find some support for the laterality hypothesis. Furthermore, those studies that looked for relationships with clinical dimensions found the effect stronger for certain subtypes.

RESULTS OF UNIVERSITY OF PENNSYLVANIA PET STUDIES

We have examined the laterality hypothesis on an initial sample of 12 patients off medications and 12 normal control subjects, using [^{18}F]FDG (Gur et al. 1987b). Subjects were studied with eyes open and ears unoccluded. While there was no laterality × diagnosis interaction on overall hemispheric metabolism, relatively higher left hemispheric metabolism for subcortical than for cortical regions was noted, and patients with more severe psychopathology had higher left hemispheric metabolism (Figure 3-1).

In a repeated evaluation of 15 patients and 8 control subjects who were studied twice (Gur et al. 1987b), the laterality index of left-right hemispheric metabolism was found reliable with a test-retest correlation of 0.63 for patients and 0.67 for control subjects (Figure 3-2). Furthermore, change in laterality from first to second study toward lower left relative to right hemispheric metabolism correlated positively (0.52) with clinical improvement, measured by the Brief Psychiatric Rating Scale (BPRS). This is illustrated in Figure 3-3.

The results provided partial support for the hypothesis of hemispheric dysfunction in schizophrenia. No overall hemispheric differences between patients and control subjects were evident, but, within patients, higher left hemispheric activity was associated with more severe symptoms. The relationship between clinical improvement and laterality change is particularly encouraging, since it suggests that laterality may be causally related to severity of symptoms in schizophrenia. It is unlikely that such a correlation would be produced by an epiphenomenon.

The issue of relevance of the laterality measure for understanding the symptomatology of schizophrenia was examined directly in comparison with the "frontality" measure (Gur et al. 1989). The strategy we have used was to begin with the physiologic parameters and examine their relationship to symptom specificity. We defined a laterality index (left-right) and a frontality index (frontal-posterior) on the basis of the PET glucose metabolic rates in a sample of 20 patients. A symptom specificity index was derived from the BPRS by identifying items tapping symptoms more specific to schizophrenia (e.g., conceptual disorganization, hallucinatory behavior, unusual thought content, blunted affect) and subtracting the average ratings on these items from the average of the nonspecific items. As can be seen in Figure 3-4, the laterality index correlated positively with symptom specificity, whereas the frontality index did not.

It is noteworthy that nearly identical effects were found with another sample we have studied with the 133-xenon inhalation technique for measuring CBF (Gur et al. 1985a).

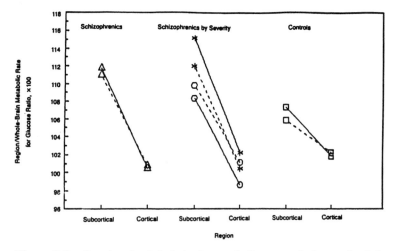

Figure 3-1.   Local-region/whole-brain metabolic rates of glucose for left (*solid lines*) and right (*broken lines*) hemispheres in cortical and subcortical regions for entire sample of schizophrenic patients, those with high (*asterisks*) and low (*circles*) severity, and control subjects. Reprinted with permission from Gur RE, Resnick SM, Alavi A, et al: Regional brain function in schizophrenia, I: a positron emission tomography study. Arch Gen Psychiatry 44:119–125, 1987. Copyright 1987 American Medical Association.

We have now completed the study of 64 subjects (32 patients with schizophrenia and 32 normal control subjects) on the PET-V device, a scanner with a spatial resolution of 17 mm full width, half maximum. These data are being analyzed. Preliminary analyses indicate that the laterality effects are maintained in this larger sample, with higher specificity of symptoms associated with relatively higher left hemispheric metabolism.

CONCLUSIONS

A search for neurophysiologic substrates of functional brain asymmetry can be helpful for understanding the neural basis of behavior and psychopathology. Hemispheric asymmetry is admittedly only one dimension, and many others can be constructed and evaluated. However, it is an important dimension neurobehaviorally in view of the vast literature on hemispheric specialization of brain function. Establishing the lateralized dysfunction of schizophrenia can place this disorder in the context of other brain diseases and suggest mechanisms for pathophysiology and perhaps treatment. PET re-

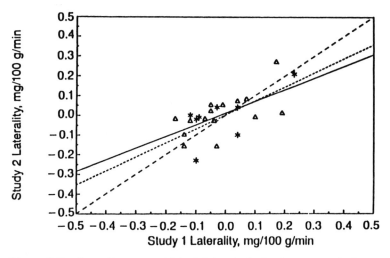

Figure 3-2. Laterality scores (right-left hemispheric glucose metabolism) for study 1 and study 2 of Gur et al. 1987. Schizophrenic patients: *triangles, solid line*; $r(13) = .63$, $P < .05$. Control subjects: *asterisks, short dotted line*; $r(6) = .67$, $P < .05$. Reprinted with permission from Gur RE, Resnick SM, Gur RC, et al: Regional brain function in schizophrenia, II: repeated evaluation with positron emission tomography. Arch Gen Psychiatry 44:126–129, 1987. Copyright 1987 American Medical Association.

search is more likely to benefit when integrated with clinical data and focused on hypotheses derived from advances in the neurobehavioral sciences. Schizophrenia is not a frontal lobe disease or a left hemispheric disease. Rather, disturbances in these and other dimensions can help explain its complex presentation and course, and variations on such dimensions can be related to clinical variability.

With these considerations in mind, we believe there is converging evidence for lateralized brain disturbance in some forms of schizophrenia. The PET studies appear to show consistently that when abnormal laterality is observed, the left hemisphere has higher metabolism, particularly in more severely disturbed patients. Our findings on correlations with symptom specificity should be pursued further, and we hope that other centers will examine this issue.

Thus far, the interpretation of PET results has been done without the benefit of integrating neuroanatomic findings. This is another important limitation, since reduced metabolic rate in patients with

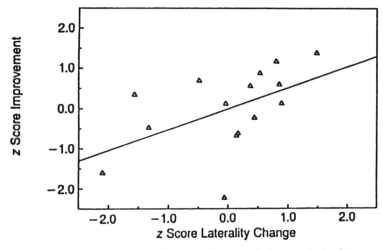

Figure 3-3. Change in laterality scores from study 1 to study 2 of Gur et al. 1987, plotted against clinical improvement. Laterality change = study 2 right-left hemispheric metabolism − study 1 right-left hemispheric metabolism. Improvement = (BPRS study 1 − BPRS study 2)/BPRS study 1, where BPRS represents Brief Psychiatric Rating Scale. Relative right hemispheric increase from study 1 to study 2 is associated with greater improvement; $r(13) = .52$, $P < .05$. Reprinted with permission from Gur RE, Resnick SM, Gur RC, et al: Regional brain function in schizophrenia; II: repeated evaluation with positron emission tomography. Arch Gen Psychiatry 44:126–129, 1987. Copyright 1987 American Medical Association.

schizophrenia could be secondary to neuronal loss. There is an increasing body of evidence that schizophrenia is associated with increased atrophic signs and, since PET integrates data across regions that may have significant atrophy, any global or regional hypometabolism could reflect the inclusion of cerebrospinal fluid in the analysis. Work is currently under way in several centers to permit correction of metabolic values derived by PET for atrophy data obtained by computed tomography or magnetic resonance imaging on the same subjects. Such studies could also help better define the anatomic location of metabolic changes.

On the other hand, it is important to recognize that these effects with PET are not isolated findings. They are consistent with a considerable body of neurobehavioral, neuroanatomic, and neurophysiologic evidence obtained with other techniques that implicate left hemispheric dysfunction in schizophrenic patients, most evident in the temporal lobe. Future studies would do well to attempt an integration of PET data with neuroanatomic and neurobehavioral data to achieve a more coherent understanding of how brain behavior relations are instrumental in giving rise to the phenomenology of

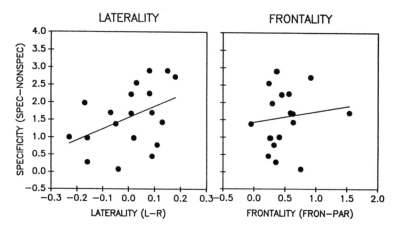

Figure 3-4. Scatterplots and regression lines showing the relation between the symptom specificity index and cerebral metabolic rate (CMR) laterality and frontality scores. Correlations are .44 ($P < .05$) for laterality and .12 (NS) for frontality. Units for CMR are mg/100 g/min. Reprinted with permission from Gur RE, Resnick SM, Gur RC: Laterality and frontality of cerebral blood flow and metabolism in schizophrenia: relationship to symptom specificity. Psychiatry Res 27:325–334, 1989. Copyright 1989 Elsevier Scientific Publishers.

schizophrenia. We think that the most fruitful avenue would be to examine subtypes of patients and to go beyond resting measures by applying the cognitive activation "challenge" paradigms we (Gur et al. 1983, 1985, 1987a) and others (Weinberger et al. 1986) have used with other neurophysiologic techniques. In schizophrenia, as with other brain disorders including stroke (Gur et al. 1988), activated measures may reveal abnormalities that are not apparent in the resting state. With carefully designed activation procedures it would be possible not only to identify such abnormalities, but also to relate them systematically to behavioral dimensions central to the psychopathology of schizophrenia.

REFERENCES

Buchsbaum MS, Ingvar DH, Kessler R, et al: Cerebral glucography with positron tomography. Arch Gen Psychiatry 39:251–259, 1982

Buchsbaum MS, Ingvar DH, Kessler R, et al: Anteroposterior gradients in cerebral glucose use in schizophrenia and affective disorder. Arch Gen Psychiatry 41:1159–1166, 1984

Cleghorn JM, Garnett ES, Nahmias C, et al: Increased frontal and reduced parietal glucose metabolism in acute untreated schizophrenia. Psychiatry Res 28:119–133, 1989

DeLisi LE, Holcomb HH, Cohen RM, et al: Positron emission tomography in schizophrenic patients with and without neuroleptic medication. J Cereb Blood Flow Metab 5:201–206, 1985

DeLisi LE, Buchsbaum MS, Holcomb HH, et al: Increased temporal lobe glucose use in chronic schizophrenic patients. Biol Psychiatry 25:835–851, 1989

Early TS, Reiman EM, Raichle ME, et al: Left globus pallidus abnormality in never-medicated patients with schizophrenia. Proc Natl Acad Sci USA 84:561–563, 1987

Farde L, Wiesel FA, Hall H, et al: No D_2 receptor increase in PET study of schizophrenia. Arch Gen Psychiatry 44:671–672, 1987

Flor-Henry P, Fromm-Auch D, Schopflocher D: Neuropsychological dimensions in psychopathology, in Laterality and Psychopathology. Amsterdam, Elsevier Biomedical, 1983

Gur RE: Left hemisphere dysfunction and left hemisphere overactivation in schizophrenia. J Abnorm Psychol 87:226–238, 1978

Gur RE: Hemispheric activation in schizophrenia: regional cerebral blood flow, in Lateralization and Psychopathology. Edited by Flor-Henry P, Gruzelier J. Amsterdam, Elsevier Biomedical, 1983

Gur RC, Reivich M: Cognitive task effects on hemispheric blood flow in humans: evidence for individual differences in hemispheric activation. Brain Lang 9:78–92, 1980

Gur RC, Gur RE, Obrist WD, et al: Sex and handedness differences in cerebral blood flow during rest and cognitive activity. Science 217:659–661, 1982

Gur RC, Gur RE, Skolnick BE, et al: Effects of task difficulty on regional cerebral blood flow: relationships with anxiety and performance. Psychophysiology 25:392–399, 1988

Gur RE, Skolnick BE, Gur RC, et al: Brain function in psychiatric disorders, I: regional cerebral blood flow in medicated schizophrenics. Arch Gen Psychiatry 40:1250–1254, 1983

Gur RE, Gur RC, Skolnick BE, et al: Brain function in psychiatric disorders, III: regional cerebral blood flow in unmedicated schizophrenics. Arch Gen Psychiatry 42:329–334, 1985

Gur RE, Resnick SM, Alavi A, et al: Regional brain function in schizophrenia, I: a positron emission tomography study. Arch Gen Psychiatry 44:119–125, 1987a

Gur RE, Resnick SM, Gur RC, et al: Regional brain function in schizophrenia, II: repeated evaluation with positron emission tomography. Arch Gen Psychiatry 44:126–129, 1987b

Gur RE, Resnick SM, Gur RC: Laterality and frontality of cerebral blood flow and metabolism in schizophrenia: relationship to symptom specificity. Psychiatry Res 27:325–334, 1989

Kimura D, Milner B: Brain mechanisms suggested by studies of temporal lobes, in Brain Underlying Speech and Language. Edited by Millikan CH, Darley FL. New York, Grune & Stratton, 1967

Sheppard G, Gruzelier J, Manchanda R, et al: ^{15}O positron emission tomographic scanning in predominantly never-treated acute schizophrenic patients. Lancet 2:1448–1452, 1983

Szechtman H, Nahmias C, Garnett S, et al: Effect of neuroleptics on altered cerebral glucose metabolism in schizophrenia. Arch Gen Psychiatry 45:523–532, 1988

Volkow ND, Brodie JD, Wolf AP, et al: Brain organization in schizophrenia. J Cereb Blood Flow Metab 6:441–446, 1986a

Volkow ND, Brodie JD, Wolf AP, et al: Brain metabolism in patients with schizophrenia before and after acute neuroleptic administration. J Neurol Neurosurg Psychiatry 49:1199–1202, 1986b

Volkow ND, Wolf AP, Van Gelder P, et al: Phenomenological correlates of metabolic activity in 18 patients with chronic schizophrenia. Am J Psychiatry 14:151–158, 1987

Weinberger DR, Berman KF, Zec RF: Physiologic dysfunction of dorsolateral prefrontal cortex in schizophrenia, I: regional cerebral blood flow evidence. Arch Gen Psychiatry 43:114–124, 1986

Wiesel FA, Wik G, Blomqvist SG, et al: Regional brain glucose metabolism in drug free schizophrenic patients and clinical correlates. Acta Psychiatr Scand 76:628–641, 1987

Wik G, Wiesel FA, Sjogren I, et al: Effects of sulpiride and chlorpromazine on regional cerebral glucose metabolism in schizophrenic patients as determined by positron emission tomography. Psychopharmacology 97:309–318, 1989

Chapter 4

Clinical Interpretation of Metabolic and Neurochemical Abnormalities in Schizophrenic Patients Studied With Positron-Emission Tomography

Nora D. Volkow, M.D., Alfred P. Wolf, Ph.D.,
Jonathan D. Brodie, M.D., Ph.D., and
Robert Cancro, M.D.

The studies done with positron-emission tomography (PET) in schizophrenic patients can be broadly divided into two categories: metabolic studies and neuroreceptor studies. Within the metabolic studies several findings have been generated that have in turn provoked controversy and formulated new questions. Among them are the following:

1. A number of studies have reported metabolic hypofrontality in schizophrenic patients. What is the significance of the findings? Is this a state or a trait characteristic of the disease? Is it a consequence of the disease or a consequence of years of neuroleptic treatment? Is it specific for schizophrenia or can it be seen in other psychiatric disorders? What is the relation between the clinical characteristics of the patients and the decrease in metabolism of the frontal cortex? How does decreased metabolism in the frontal cortex affect the overall function of other brain areas with which the frontal cortex has important connections?

2. Increased metabolism in the basal ganglia has been reported in schizophrenic patients. What is the significance of this finding? Is this finding related to the clinical syndrome or a consequence of chronic neuroleptic treatment? Are the metabolic changes specific

This research was supported under Contract No. DE-AC02-76CH00016 with the U.S. Department of Energy and NIH Grant 15380.

for schizophrenia or do they exist in other types of psychotic disorders?

3. How do the PET findings have an impact on our notions of the schizophrenic process? Do they corroborate the laterality hypothesis of schizophrenia? Is there evidence of homogeneous or heterogeneous patterns of abnormal metabolism in the brain of schizophrenic patients that would support either the homogeneous or heterogeneous definition of schizophrenia? Is there evidence of a localized instead of a widespread pattern of abnormalities in the brain of schizophrenic patients?

Receptor studies using PET have focused mainly on the investigation of dopamine receptors in the brains of schizophrenic subjects. As will be described in more detail in the next chapters in this book, major emphasis has been placed on determining whether schizophrenic patients have an abnormal number of dopamine receptors as well as on finding an optimal tracer to monitor the number of dopamine receptors in the brains of individuals. In this chapter, we focus on those strategies that may help resolve some clinical questions about schizophrenia. More specifically, does the plasma concentration of the neuroleptic reflect the actual amount of neuroleptic that goes into the brain and binds to the receptor? Is there a relationship between the clinical response of the schizophrenic patient to the neuroleptic and the percentage of receptors blocked by the neuroleptic? Can schizophrenic patients who are responders be distinguished from those who are nonresponders on the basis of receptor number or properties?

In this chapter we review some of the answers that have been given to these questions.

METABOLIC STUDIES

Studies measuring regional brain metabolism in schizophrenic patients have been done with different tracers: ^{18}F-labeled fluorodeoxyglucose ($[^{18}$F]FDG) and ^{11}C-labeled deoxyglucose to measure regional glucose metabolism (Reivich et al. 1985), and ^{15}O-labeled oxygen to measure oxygen metabolism.

Hypofrontality

Decreased metabolic activity of the frontal cortex was the first abnormality reported in schizophrenic patients using PET (Farkas et al. 1980). Since then several papers have replicated these findings (Buchsbaum et al. 1982, 1984; Farkas et al. 1984; Volkow et al. 1986a; Wolkin et al. 1985, 1988). However, there has also been a series of studies failing to show decreased metabolic activity in the brains of schizophrenic patients (Early et al. 1987; Gur et al. 1987; Sheppard et al. 1983; Volkow et al. 1986b; Widen et al. 1983). The lack of reproducibility of the hypofrontality by some investigators could be addressed as representing either differences in the methodology employed to study these patients or differences in the patient populations investigated. Among the latter there has been an interest in determining whether the clinical characteristics of the patient affect the presence of hypofrontality or whether hypofrontality occurs at a certain stage during the disease.

Differences in the clinical characteristics of the patients as well as staging of the disease are of importance in order to interpret the PET findings. Most of the studies that have failed to report hypofrontality have been done in schizophrenic patients who have an acute presentation of their illness at the time of the study (Early et al. 1987; Sheppard et al. 1983; Volkow et al. 1986b), in contrast to the studies that have reported hypofrontality that were done mainly in chronic patients (Buchsbaum et al. 1982, 1984; Farkas et al. 1984; Volkow et al. 1986a; Wolkin et al. 1985, 1988). To further investigate this issue, we analyzed the metabolic PET images in a group of 18 chronic schizophrenic patients to determine if degree of chronicity was related to degree of hypofrontality. We found that the hypofrontality correlated significantly with the age of the patients, with years of illness, and with clinical presentation. Hypofrontality was seen in those patients showing a deficit state as assessed by the presence of negative symptoms. It was the relation between age and severity of negative symptoms that correlated with hypofrontality (Volkow et al. 1987a). We were unable to show hypofrontality in younger patients with short illness duration and with low grading in negative symptoms. The association between negative symptoms and hypofrontality was accentuated when testing the schizophrenic subject with a task that activated the frontal cortex, since these patients failed to activate the frontal cortex in response to the task. Although these findings corroborate some relationship between the clinical characteristics of the patient and the decreased metabolic activity of the frontal cortex, we cannot rule out the contribution of chronic neuroleptic treatment to the decreased metabolism of the frontal cortex seen in chronic schizophrenic patients. This is relevant, since studies done on patients who had received minimal or no neuroleptic exposure failed to show hypofrontality (Early et al. 1987; Volkow et al. 1986b).

Another way to assess the contribution of neuroleptic treatment to hypofrontality has been to measure regional brain glucose metabolism in schizophrenic patients before and after treatment with neuroleptics until clinical response. These studies reported that chronic neuroleptic treatment increases brain glucose metabolism with a relatively smaller change in the frontal cortex, thus accentuating the hypofrontality observed initially in these patients (DeLisi et al. 1985; Wolkin et al. 1985). The above studies suggest that the hypofrontality seen in the schizophrenic subjects is not a trait of the disease but is probably due to chronic neuroleptics and the aging process in these patients. It may be that the pattern of hypofrontality represents an end stage of the disease that appears clinically as a deficiency state.

The specificity of the findings of hypofrontality in the schizophrenic patients has also been questioned inasmuch as decreased metabolic activity in the frontal cortex has also been reported to occur in patients with affective disorders (Baxter et al. 1985; Buchsbaum et al. 1984; Volkow et al. 1988c) and with chronic cocaine abuse (Volkow et al. 1988d).

The frontal cortex is highly interconnected with cortical, subcortical, and limbic areas and has been postulated to play a key role in regulating brain activities (Stuss and Benson 1986). Hence, disruptions of the frontal lobe should be expected to indirectly disturb activity of other brain areas. Some preliminary attempts have been made to investigate the effect of decreased frontal activity in the overall pattern of organization of the brain of schizophrenic patients. One approach has been to investigate the pattern of association among major brain areas using the correlation coefficients among regional metabolic values (Horwitz et al. 1984). This approach is based on the hypothesis that measurement of covariation between pairs of brain regions reflects the functional relationship between them. These studies have revealed decreased correlations among brain areas of schizophrenic subjects when compared with normal subjects (Clark et al. 1984; Volkow et al. 1988a), a pattern characterized mainly by decreased interactions between the anterior and posterior areas of the brain. Another interesting finding of these studies has been that the pattern of interactions among brain areas of the schizophrenic individual's brain changes less than that of the brain of a normal individual when receiving an external stimulation (Volkow et al. 1988a). Decreased ability to respond to external stimulation could result from decreased function of the frontal cortex, since this is an area of the brain that modulates and integrates external stimuli (Luria 1980).

Subcortical Abnormalities

The advent of PET allowed for the first time noninvasive investigation of the biochemistry and metabolism of subcortical structures in human subjects. The studies conducted in chronic schizophrenic patients and acute schizophrenic patients have reported increased metabolic activity in the basal ganglia of schizophrenic patients when compared with normal subjects (Early et al. 1987; Gur et al. 1987; Volkow et al. 1986a, 1986b). Increased metabolic activity of the basal ganglia has been reported in patients who have never received neuroleptic treatment and in those who have a long history of neuroleptic exposure, as well as in patients with and without decreased metabolic activity of the frontal cortex. Demonstration of abnormalities in the basal ganglia of schizophrenic patients is of interest because of the traditional implications that the therapeutic efficacy of neuroleptics is due to their action on the mesolimbic dopamine system and that the action of neuroleptics on the nigrostriatal system is responsible for the extrapyramidal side effects of these drugs (Snyder et al. 1974; Van Pragg 1977). This view is now being further challenged by new studies that show that the basal ganglia are responsible not only for motor function but for memory and other functions, such as modulation of sensory input, attention, neuronal, memory, and higher cognitive functions (Hassler 1977). Since subcortical structures have multiple connections with cortex and limbic structures (Schneider 1984), their dysfunction could affect several cerebral systems. Abnormalities of basal ganglia function as a primary defect in schizophrenia have been postulated by previous investigators as a possible factor in the dysfunctions in schizophrenic patients (Lidsky et al. 1979).

Metabolic abnormalities in the basal ganglia, however, do not appear to be unique to schizophrenia and have been reported in other types of patients. More specifically, we have shown increased metabolic activity of the basal ganglia in patients with systemic lupus erythematosus who were psychotic at the time of the study (Volkow et al. 1988b) as well as in an AIDS patient who was catatonic at the time of the PET scan (Volkow et al. 1987b). As in the case of hypofrontality, metabolic changes in the basal ganglia do not appear to be specific to schizophrenia.

Abnormalities in Other Brain Areas

Metabolic abnormalities have also been described for other brain areas in schizophrenic subjects. Decreased metabolism in the parietal cortex has been reported to occur in acute and chronic schizophrenic patients (Kishimoto et al. 1987; Wiesel et al. 1987). Increased metabolism of the temporal lobes has been reported in schizophrenic subjects. The increased metabolism in the temporal cortex was greater in the left hemisphere (DeLisi et al. 1985). The latter findings are of relevance because they also touch on the "laterality" theory of schizophrenia, namely, that schizophrenic patients have abnormal left hemisphere function (Flor-Henry and Gruzelier 1983). The PET studies trying to document laterality have been controversial. In support of this theory, there have been some studies documenting increased metabolism in the left hemisphere of schizophrenic patients (Gur et al. 1987; Sheppard et al. 1983). However, most of the studies have failed to show a clear pattern of asymmetries in the brains of schizophrenic patients. Although we were unable in our studies to document a specific pattern of lateralization in schizophrenia, we showed that clinical symptoms were related to regional brain abnormalities of the left hemisphere with more frequency than with the right hemisphere (Volkow et al. 1987a).

An area of controversy in schizophrenic research is whether schizophrenia represents one disorder (homogeneous) or is, in fact, a set of disorders (heterogeneous) (Bleuler 1950; Cancro 1970; Ciompi 1984). Although there has not been a sufficient number of studies done with PET in schizophrenic patients to ascertain whether there are subgroups of schizophrenic individuals that can be characterized by specific patterns of brain metabolism, there have been two studies that suggest that the metabolic abnormalities are not the same across groups of schizophrenic patients. One study documents differences in brain metabolism between schizophrenic subjects with "predominantly negative symptoms" and schizophrenic patients with "predominantly positive symptoms" (Volkow et al. 1987a). Another study reported three subgroups of schizophrenic patients based on the pattern of metabolic abnormalities: one with decreased metabolism of the frontal cortex, a second with decreased metabolism of the parietal cortex, and a third with a "normal" metabolic pattern (Kishimoto et al. 1987). Unfortunately, there are not yet enough normative data to assess whether subgroups of metabolic patterns also exist in normal subjects. Until this information exists and until more schizophrenic patients have been investigated, we will not be able to interpret the pathophysiological significance of these metabolic patterns.

As is clear from the previous discussion, PET studies with currently available labeled probes have failed to reveal a consistent, well-localized area of abnormality in the brain of schizophrenic patients. Although lack of agreement could well represent methodological differences among investigators, it could also represent that fact that deficits in the brain of schizophrenic patients may not be well localized but rather represent a more widespread pattern of derangements that involve several brain structures. As discussed earlier, this should be expected if, in fact, there are abnormalities in the frontal cortex and basal ganglia of schizophrenic patients, since these areas are highly connected with the rest of the brain. To assess whether metabolic patterns could be found that were different in schizophrenic patients beyond the abnormalities in the frontal cortex and basal ganglia, we analyzed the brain as a whole in normal subjects and schizophrenic patients. Metabolic differences among both groups were apparent across all brain levels analyzed and revealed that normal subjects have higher levels of activity in anterior and superior areas of the brain than schizophrenic patients (Levy et al. 1989).

Although no definitive questions have yet been answered on metabolic abnormalities in schizophrenic patients, the knowledge and methodology are evolving. It is hoped that it will help us to better understand the pathophysiological mechanism of schizophrenia.

Lessons to be learned from 10 years of investigating metabolic abnormalities in schizophrenic patients are the importance of adequate definition of the clinical characteristics of the patient to be studied, the influence of such variables as neuroleptics and age on regional brain glucose metabolism, the importance of analyzing the brain as an integrated unit in contrast to multiple isolated brain regions, and the utility of designing strategies to activate specific areas of the brain to accentuate abnormal patterns of function and interaction.

RECEPTOR STUDIES

Most of the PET studies done to evaluate receptors in schizophrenic patients have focused on the dopamine receptors. Several tracers have been proposed to measure dopamine receptors with PET, such as ^{18}F-labeled *N*-methylspiroperidol (^{18}F-NMS; Arnett 1985), ^{11}C-labeled raclopride (Farde et al. 1986), and [76]Br-labeled bromospiperone ([[76]Br]BSP; Baron et al. 1986). The latter compounds have been used to label the dopamine postsynaptic receptors. The characteristics of these compounds and the mathematical models employed in their analyses are reviewed in Chapter 6. In this chapter we only review their clinical applications in the area of schizophrenia.

Concentration of Dopamine Receptors in Schizophrenic Patients

Postmortem studies have revealed a higher density of dopamine receptors in the striatum of some schizophrenic patients than in the striatum of normal subjects. Elevated dopamine receptor densities are reported to occur both in chronically treated and in never-medicated schizophrenic patients (Seeman et al. 1987). With PET and an appropriate model, one can evaluate some properties of dopamine receptors in the brain of living schizophrenic patients (Wagner et al.

1984). So far, results obtained with PET have been controversial, with one group reporting a twofold to threefold elevation of D_2 receptors in the basal ganglia of 10 never-medicated and 5 previously medicated schizophrenic patients (Wong et al. 1986) and another group failing to find an increase in dopamine receptor density in the basal ganglia of schizophrenic patients (Farde et al. 1987). The discrepancy in the results has not yet been resolved and could be accounted for by methodological differences among investigators and/or differences in patient populations. These possibilities are addressed in greater detail in Chapter 6.

The specificity of the finding of increased dopamine receptors in the basal ganglia of some schizophrenic patients has been challenged by similar increases in psychotic manic patients (Wong et al. 1988), in a nonpsychotic, never-medicated patient with methylphenyltetra-hydropyridine (MPTP)–induced parkinsonism (Perlmutter et al. 1987), and in patients with Tourette's syndrome (Wong et al. 1988). The pathological significance of changes in the number or occupancy of dopamine receptors with respect to psychoses, schizophrenia, and movement disorders has not been resolved.

Relation Between Neuroleptic Concentration in Plasma and Brain

The therapeutic efficacy of neuroleptic drugs has been related to their ability to block central dopamine receptors (Snyder et al. 1974). In fact, animal studies have shown a linear relation between the affinity of different neuroleptics for the D_2 receptor and their efficacy as antipsychotic agents in humans (Creese et al. 1976). In contrast to this linear relation between affinity for D_2 receptors and antipsychotic potency, the studies performed with humans to investigate the relation between plasma concentration of neuroleptics and their antipsychotic effects have failed to show such a clear relation (Dahl 1986). Plausible explanations include differences in metabolism and transport of neuroleptic from plasma into the brain among individuals. These notions have led clinicians to increase the dose of neuroleptics in nonresponding patients even when the patients' neuroleptic plasma levels are within "therapeutic" ranges. With PET it has been feasible to investigate the relation between plasma neuroleptic concentration and degree of occupancy of the dopamine receptors by the neuroleptic drug. This has been feasible because the neuroleptic will bind to the dopamine receptor, thus blocking its ability to bind to the positron-labeled dopamine ligand (Smith et al. 1988). Therefore, when doing a study to measure uptake of the radioactive dopamine ligand in a patient who is being treated with a neuroleptic, the amount of radioactive ligand binding to the basal ganglia will be related to the

number of free receptors. Figure 4-1 shows the images obtained with
^{18}F-NMS in a schizophrenic patient who was being treated with 10
mg of haloperidol. The upper images represent the first scan done in
this patient 2 hours after his last dose of neuroleptic. The lower images
represent the scan done 24 hours after the last dose of haloperidol.
As can be seen, there is a considerable increase in ^{18}F-NMS uptake
24 hours after the last dose of haloperidol due to a decrease in the
concentration of haloperidol in the brain, which competes for the

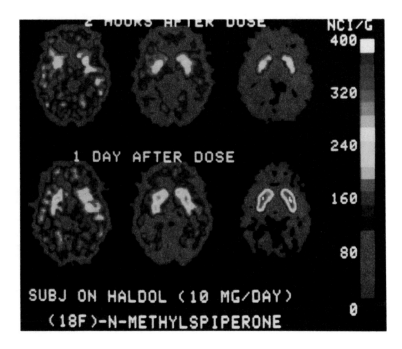

Figure 4-1. Images obtained with ^{18}F-labeled *N*-methylspiperone
(^{18}F-NMS) at the level of the basal ganglia. The images on the upper row
of the figure were taken 2 hours after haloperidol administration. The images
on the lower row were taken 24 hours after the last dose of haloperidol.
Each row shows the images obtained at 20, 120, and 240 minutes after [18]F-
NMS administration. Notice the higher uptake of ^{18}F-NMS after 24 hours
of haloperidol.

same receptor as the radioactive ligand, ^{18}F-NMS. The relation between plasma concentration of neuroleptics and binding of radioactive dopamine ligands has been studied using ^{18}F-NMS (Smith et al. 1988) and [[76]B]BSP (Cambon et al. 1987). These studies have measured the percentage of receptors blocked by different plasma concentrations of neuroleptics and have shown a curvilinear relationship between plasma level and dopamine receptor occupancy. This curve shows that small doses of neuroleptic block a proportionally higher number of dopamine receptors than the high doses. This means that in order to block 25% of the receptors, a relatively small dose of the neuroleptic is required, whereas to change the number of blocked receptors from 75% to a greater value, relatively large amounts of the neuroleptic are required. The above results document several important clinical issues, namely

1. Plasma level measurement of neuroleptics reflects receptor occupancy by neuroleptics.
2. Upper limit for neuroleptic concentration exists, after which increasing neuroleptic doses will not be of much benefit in further blocking the dopamine receptor (between 15–20 mg/ml for haloperidol).
3. Therapeutic efficacy appears to occur when 65–85% of the receptors are blocked.
4. The amount of time required for complete washout of neuroleptic from the dopamine receptors was measured to be between 5 and 12 days, which is a much shorter washout period than that determined from behavioral and pharmacokinetic data (Baldessarini et al. 1988).

Relation Between Blockade of Dopamine Receptors by Neuroleptics and Their Clinical Efficacy

Although neuroleptics have clinical efficacy for the majority of schizophrenic patients, a subgroup will show minimal or no antipsychotic response to neuroleptics. Considerable effort has been expended in trying to understand the characteristics of nonresponders and to determine whether this group of patients either represents a subgroup of schizophrenic patients with no defects in dopamine or represents different stages of the disease, or whether they are not responding because of differences in metabolism of neuroleptics. Preliminary studies have been done to answer some of these questions. These studies have examined whether there are differences in dopamine receptors between responders and nonresponders and whether there are differences in dopamine receptor blockade by neuroleptics between the responders and the nonresponders. An initial study failed to show differences in ^{18}F-NMS binding between responders and nonresponders (Wolkin et al. 1987). This study failed to report any significant differences in receptor blockade by neuroleptics between responders and nonresponders. A different study reported that all patients who had receptor blockade between 65% and 85% had a good response to neuroleptic treatment and that the patient with 86% blockade was the only one with extrapyramidal symptoms (Farde et al. 1988). These symptoms disappeared with drug reduction with no detrimental effect on the antipsychotic efficacy of the drug. Based on these results, the investigators hypothesized that a lower receptor occupancy may be required for the antipsychotic effects than the occupancy required for extrapyramidal side effects.

CONCLUSION

PET has been used over the past 10 years to try to define metabolic and neurochemical deficits in the brains of schizophrenic patients that may relate to etiopathogenesis and/or that may help better categorize these patients. Though none of these studies has yet been conclusive, they have disclosed regional cerebral functional abnormalities that have led to hypotheses about patterns of brain dysfunction in these patients. Some of these findings such as the hypofrontality and laterality have been previously reported using other techniques. Other findings, such as the abnormalities in the basal ganglia, have been disclosed for the first time in the living schizophrenic patient. Similarly, the receptor studies are allowing investigators to test previous hypotheses about neurotransmitter defects in schizophrenic patients, while at the same time the development of new tracer ligands is opening the investigation of neurotransmitters other than dopamine that may be of relevance in schizophrenic disorders and their treatment.

REFERENCES

Arnett CD, Fowler JS, Wolf AP, et al: [18]F-*N*-methylspiroperidol the radioligand of choice for PET studies of the dopamine receptor in human brain. Life Sci 36:1359–1366, 1985

Baldessarini RJ, Cohen BM, Teicher MH: Dose effect relationships of antipsychotic agents. Arch Gen Psychiatry 44:79–91, 1988

Baron J, Maziere B, Loch C, et al: Loss of striatal [76]Br-bromospiperone–binding sites demonstrated by positron tomography in progressive supranuclear palsy. J Cereb Blood Flow Metab 6:131–136, 1986

Baxter LR, Phelps ME, Mazziotta J, et al: Cerebral metabolic rates for glucose in mood disorders. Arch Gen Psychiatry 42:441–447, 1985

Bleuler E: Dementia Praecox: Or the Group of Schizophrenias. New York, International Universities Press, 1950

Buchsbaum MS, Ingvar DH, Kessler R, et al: Cerebral glucography with positron tomography. Arch Gen Psychiatry 39:252–259, 1982

Buchsbaum MS, DeLisi LE, Holcomb HH, et al: Anteroposterior gradients in cerebral glucose use in schizophrenia and affective disorders. Arch Gen Psychiatry 41:1159–1166, 1984

Cambon H, Baron JC, Boulenger JP, et al: In vivo assay for neuroleptic receptor binding in the striatum positron tomography in humans. Br J Psychiatry 151:824–830, 1987

Cancro R: A classificatory principle in schizophrenia. Am J Psychiatry 126:131–135, 1970

Ciompi L: Is there really a schizophrenia? the long-term course of psychotic phenomena. Br J Psychiatry 145:636–640, 1984

Clark CM, Kessler R, Buchsbaum MS, et al: Correlational methods for determining regional coupling of cerebral glucose metabolism: a pilot study. Biol Psychiatry 19:663–678, 1984

Creese I, Burt DR, Snyder SH: Dopamine receptor binding predicts clinical and pharmacological potencies of antischizophrenic drugs. Science 192:481–483, 1976

Dahl S: Plasma level monitoring of antipsychotic drugs: clinical utility. Clin Pharmacokinet 11:36–61, 1986

DeLisi LE, Holcomb HH, Cohen RM, et al: Positron emission tomography in schizophrenic patients with and without neuroleptic medication. J Cereb Blood Flow Metab 5:201–206, 1985

Early TS, Reiman EM, Raichle ME, et al: Left globus pallidus abnormality in never-medicated patients with schizophrenia. Proc Natl Acad Sci USA 84:561–563, 1987

Farde L, Hall H, Ehrin E, et al: Quantitative analysis of D_2 dopamine receptor binding in the human brain by PET. Science 231:258–261, 1986

Farde L, Weisel FA, Hall H, et al: No D_2 receptor increase in PET study of schizophrenia. Arch Gen Psychiatry 44:671–672, 1987

Farde L, Wiesel F, Halldin CH, et al: Central D_2 dopamine receptor occupancy in schizophrenic patients treated with antipsychotic drugs. Arch Gen Psychiatry 45:71–76, 1988

Farkas T, Reivich M, Alavi A, et al: Application of [^{18}F]2-deoxyglucose and positron emission tomography in the study of psychiatric conditions, in Cerebral Metabolism and Neural Function. Edited by Passonneau JV, Hawkins RA, List WD, et al. Baltimore, MD, Williams & Wilkins, 1980, pp 403–408

Farkas T, Wolf AP, Jaeger J, et al: Regional brain glucose metabolism in chronic schizophrenia. Arch Gen Psychiatry 41:292–300, 1984

Flor-Henry P, Gruzelier J: Laterality and Psychopathology. Amsterdam, Elsevier Biomedical, 1983

Gur RE, Resnick SM, Alavi A, et al: Regional brain function in schizophrenia: a positron emission tomography study. Arch Gen Psychiatry 44:119–125, 1987

Hassler R: Basal ganglia systems regulating mental activity. Int J Neurol 12:53–72, 1977

Horwitz B, Duara R, Rapoport S: Intercorrelations of glucose metabolic rates between brain regions: application to healthy males in a state of reduced sensory input. J Cereb Blood Flow Metab 4:484–499, 1984

Kishimoto H, Kuwahara H, Ohno S, et al: Diseases in association areas found in chronic schizophrenics using ^{11}C-glucose PET, in Cerebral Dynamics Laterality and Psychopathology. Edited by Takahashi R, Flor-Henry P, Gruzelier J, et al. New York, Elsevier, 1987

Levy AV, Brodie JD, Russell JA, et al: The metabolic centroid method for PET brain image analysis. J Cereb Blood Flow Metab 9:388–397, 1989

Lidsky TI, Weinhold PM, Levine FM: Implications of basal ganglionic dysfunction for schizophrenia. Biol Psychiatry 14:3–12, 1979

Luria AR: Higher Cortical Functions in Man. New York, Basic Books, 1980

Perlmutter JC, Kilbournne MR, Raichle ME, et al: MPTP-induced upregulation of in vivo dopaminergic radioligand-receptor binding in human. Neurology 37:1575–1579, 1987

Reivich M, Alavi A, Wolf A, et al: Glucose metabolic rate kinetic model parameter determination in humans: the lumped constants and rate constants for (^{18}F)fluorodeoxyglucose and (^{11}C)deoxyglucose. J Cereb Blood Flow Metab 5:179–192, 1985

Schneider JS: Basal ganglia role in behavior: importance of sensory gating and its relevance to psychiatry. Biol Psychiatry 19:1693–1710, 1984

Seeman P, Ulpian C, Bergeron C, et al: Bimodal distribution of dopamine receptor densities in brains of schizophrenics. Science 225:728–731, 1987

Sheppard G, Gruzelier J, Manchanda R, et al: 15-0 positron emission tomography scanning in predominantly never-treated acute schizophrenic patients. Lancet 2:1448–1452, 1983

Smith M, Wolf AP, Brodie JD, et al: Serial ^{18}F-N-methylspiroperidol PET studies to measure changes in antipsychotic drug D$_2$ receptor occupancy in schizophrenic patients. Biol Psychiatry 23:653–663, 1988

Snyder SH, Banerjee SP, Yamamura HI, et al: Drugs, neurotransmitters and schizophrenia. Science 184:1243–1253, 1974

Stuss DT, Benson FD: The Frontal Lobes. New York, Raven, 1986

Van Pragg HM: The significance of dopamine for the mode of action of neuroleptics and the pathogenesis of schizophrenia. Br J Psychiatry 130:463–474, 1977

Volkow ND, Brodie JD, Wolf AP, et al: Brain organization in schizophrenia. J Cereb Blood Flow Metab 6:441–446, 1986a

Volkow ND, Brodie JD, Wolf AP, et al: Brain metabolism in predominantly never-treated schizophrenics before and after acute neuroleptic administration. J Neurol Neurosurg Psychiatry 49:1199–1201, 1986b

Volkow ND, Van Gelder P, Wolf AP, et al: Phenomenological correlates of metabolic activity in chronic schizophrenics. Am J Psychiatry 144:151–158, 1987a

Volkow N, Harper A, Monisteri D, et al: AIDS and catatonia. J Neurol Neurosurg Psychiatry 50:104–105, 1987b

Volkow ND, Brodie JD, Wolf AP, et al: Interactions in schizophrenics under resting and activation conditions. Schizophr Res 1:47–53, 1988a

Volkow N, Warner N, MacIntyre R, et al: Cerebral involvement in systemic lupus erythematosus. American Journal of Physiological Imaging 3:91–98, 1988b

Volkow ND, Bellar S, Mullani N, et al: Effects of electroshock on brain glucose metabolism. Convulsive Therapy 4:199–206, 1988c

Volkow ND, Mullani N, Gould L, et al: Cerebral blood flow in chronic cocaine users. Br J Psychiatry 152:641–648, 1988d

Wagner HN, Burns D, Dannals RT, et al: Imaging dopamine receptors in the human brain by positron tomography. Science 221:1264–1266, 1984

Widen L, Blomqvist G, Greitz T, et al: PET studies of glucose metabolism in patients with schizophrenia. AJNR 4:550–552, 1983

Wiesel FA, Wik G, Sjogren I, et al: Regional brain glucose metabolism in drug-free schizophrenic patients and clinical correlates. Acta Psychiatr Scand 76:628–641, 1987

Wolkin A, Jaeger J, Brodie JD, et al: Persistence of cerebral metabolic abnormalities in chronic schizophrenia as determined by positron emission tomography. Am J Psychiatry 142:564–571, 1985

Wolkin A, Barouche F, Wolf AP, et al: Dopamine blockade and clinical response: evidence for two biological subgroups of schizophrenia (abstract). Presented at the 26th annual meeting of the American College of Neuropsychopharmacology, December 1987

Wolkin A, Angrist B, Wolf AP, et al: Low frontal glucose utilization in chronic schizophrenia: a replication study. Am J Psychiatry 145:251–253, 1988

Wong DF, Wagner HN, Tune LE: Positron emission tomography reveals elevated D_2 dopamine receptors in drug-naive schizophrenics. Science 234:1558–1563, 1986

Wong DF, Singer H, Pearlson G, et al: D_2 dopamine receptors in Tourette's syndrome and manic depressive illness. J Nucl Med 29:820–821, 1988

Chapter 5

The Use of Positron-Emission Tomography in Identifying and Quantitating Receptors Involved in Schizophrenia

David J. Schlyer, Ph.D.

S chizophrenia is a devastating mental disorder that is the focus of a great deal of research. Some symptoms of the disease, such as auditory hallucinations and delusions, can be ameliorated with drug treatment, whereas other symptoms, such as social withdrawal and cognitive decline, remain uncontrolled. It is possible that these latter symptoms that are often termed "negative symptoms" are the result of anatomical and neurochemical abnormalities, whereas those symptoms of the disease such as auditory hallucinations that are termed "positive symptoms" may be a result of only neurochemical disorders (Crow 1986; Trimble 1987; Weinberger 1988a).

The drugs used to treat schizophrenia are designated neuroleptics. The term *neuroleptic* was chosen to emphasize the similarity of pharmacological profiles of drugs with entirely different chemical structures (Carlsson 1978). Especially prominent features of the effects of neuroleptics include the following: a state of affective indifference; a decrease in locomotor activity; a decrease in excitation, agitation, and aggressiveness; and an antipsychotic action in patients with acute as well as chronic psychoses.

AFFINITY VERSUS EFFICACY

Since the first use of neuroleptics for the treatment of schizophrenia in 1952 (Delay et al. 1952), there has been growing evidence that the antipsychotic drugs exert their influence at least in part by reducing dopaminergic neuronal activity mediated by the D_2 receptor (Seeman

This research was carried out at Brookhaven National Laboratory under Contract No. DE-AC2-76CH00016 with the U.S. Department of Energy and supported by NIH Grants 15638 and 15380.

1981, 1987). The dopamine hypothesis is widely accepted in explaining the neuropharmacological abnormalities that occur in schizophrenia. The central tenet of the hypothesis is that people who have the disease have an apparent hyperactivity of the dopaminergic mechanisms in critical brain regions. There are several lines of evidence to support this hypothesis, and these have been outlined by Seeman (1987). They are

1. The clinical side effects of the neuroleptics
2. The psychotomimetic effects of dopamine-mimetic drugs
3. Neuroleptic acceleration of catecholamine turnover
4. Antipsychotic potency correlates with D_2 blockade in responders
5. Elevated density of D_2 receptors in schizophrenia.

By far the most convincing of these observations is the correlation of clinical antipsychotic potency of these drugs with the affinity of the drug for the D_2 receptor. The correlation between the clinically efficient dose and the binding affinity of the neuroleptic drugs for D_2 receptors is given in Figure 5-1 (data from Closse 1984; Peroutka and

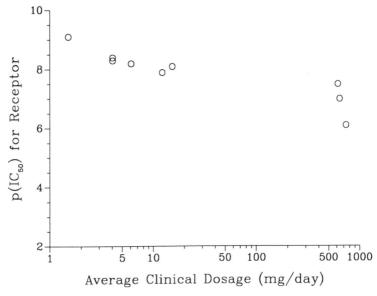

Figure 5-1. Plot of the affinity of common neuroleptic drugs for the D_2 receptor with the typical clinical dosage. Clinical dosages taken from Peroutka and Snyder 1980. Values for the $p(IC_{50})$'s taken from Closse et al. 1984.

Snyder 1980). This correlation can be compared with the correlation with other receptor subtypes. The plot of the affinity for the D_1 receptor is given in Figure 5-2. There is no correlation with this site. The similar plot for serotonin receptors is given in Figure 5-3. The plot of the affinity for the muscarinic receptor in Figure 5-4 shows a slight inverse correlation with the clinical dose. Figure 5-5 shows the plot for the sigma receptor that demonstrates no correlation between clinical dose and receptor affinity (Closse 1984; Peroutka 1980). The sigma receptor was initially thought to represent a subtype of the opiate receptors. However, the inability to block the behavioral effects of sigma drugs with naloxone and the opposite stereospecificity of opiate and sigma drugs gave evidence that the sigma receptor is different from the opiate receptor. The moderate potency of sigma drugs on phencyclidine (PCP) receptors then led to the belief that the PCP receptor mediated the action of sigma drugs (Snyder and Largent 1989). Sigma receptors are now classified as a separate receptor type. The high affinity of haloperidol to sigma receptors has generated interest with respect to their role in psychoses.

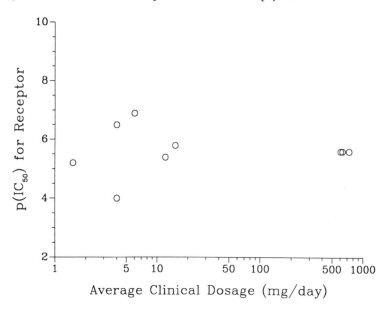

Figure 5-2. Plot of the affinity of the common neuroleptic drugs for the D_1 receptor with the typical clinical dosage. Clinical dosages taken from Peroutka and Snyder 1980. Values for the $p(IC_{50})$'s taken from Closse et al. 1984.

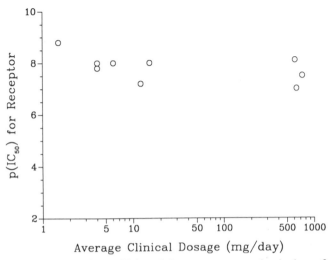

Figure 5-3.　Plot of the affinity of the common neuroleptic drugs for the serotonin receptors with the typical clinical dosage. Clinical dosages taken from Peroutka and Snyder 1980. Values for the $p(IC_{50})$'s taken from Closse et al. 1984.

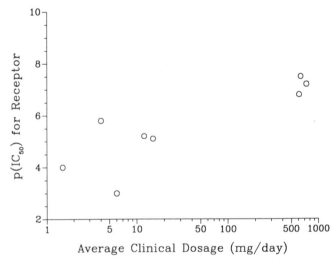

Figure 5-4.　Plot of the affinity of the common neuroleptic drugs for the muscarinic receptors with the typical clinical dosage. Clinical dosages taken from Peroutka and Snyder 1980. Values for the $p(IC_{50})$'s taken from Closse et al. 1984.

POSTMORTEM STUDIES

Postmortem studies of schizophrenic patients have shown that the D_2 receptor level was elevated in some subjects in this group (Seeman 1984). There was a bimodal distribution of receptor densities, one mode of which was significantly higher than the normal control group. The question that immediately arose was whether this elevation was due to the disease or resulted from the chronic use of neuroleptic drugs. It has been shown in animals that prolonged blockade of D_2 receptors elevates the number of receptors by approximately 30% (Seeman 1987). A study of postmortem brains of schizophrenic patients on haloperidol therapy in comparison with those who had been off drugs for 3 months and normal control subjects demonstrated a significant increase in D_2 receptor number only in those patients who were on neuroleptics at the time of death (Kornhuber et al. 1989b). Positron-emission tomography (PET) has the ability to ascertain the answer to this question directly because it is, in principle, possible to obtain information that may be used to determine the number of receptors available for binding.

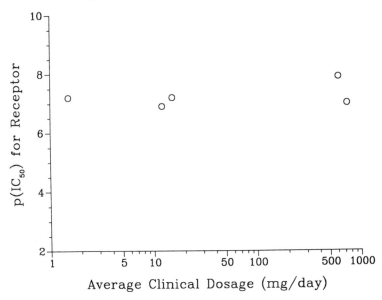

Figure 5-5. Plot of the affinity of the common neuroleptic drugs for the sigma receptors with the typical clinical dosage. Clinical dosages taken from Peroutka and Snyder 1980. Values for the $p(IC_{50})$'s taken from Closse et al. 1984.

PET STUDIES

PET is the only technique available at present that can accurately quantitate the receptor density in the living human brain, and several studies have been carried out in an attempt to accomplish this feat. There is a considerable amount of controversy at present as to the best technique to use to measure this receptor density, but there seems to be general agreement within the field that PET can be used to quantify receptor density in the living human brain once the intricacies of the experiment are understood. The controversy in general revolves around the choice of radiolabeled ligand used to measure receptor density. Some groups promote the use of low-affinity ligands that give dynamic information about the receptor availability, and other groups promote the use of very high-affinity ligands that are not displaced by endogenous ligands. These two techniques should in theory give the same results, but in fact they do not (Andreasen 1988). The explanation of these discrepancies must await further experimentation.

Another observation that requires further investigation is that in most patients, the symptoms of schizophrenia are decreased only after several weeks of treatment with neuroleptics. This corresponds to a fall in the homovanillic acid (HVA) concentration after the initial increase observed when neuroleptic therapy is begun. PET may be able to shed light on this phenomenon as one is able to correlate plasma drug levels with the receptor availability. Some work has been carried out that shows a good correlation between the receptor occupancy and the plasma level of the drug (Cambon et al. 1987; Smith et al. 1988; Wolkin et al. 1989).

The definitive test of the dopamine hypothesis of schizophrenia must also await a better understanding of the involvement of other receptor systems in the disease. It is not clear at this point in time whether the dopamine system is the only neurotransmitter system involved in the disease or whether there are several systems involved. This latter possibility seems more likely in view of the feedback loops known to exist between the dopamine system and other receptor systems (Vinick and Heym 1987). Compounds acting at sigma sites, for example, can alter dopaminergic function in the absence of direct interactions with the dopamine receptors. Some of the most effective "atypical" neuroleptics act at the sigma sites, as do some of the typical neuroleptics such as haloperidol, which binds to both D_2 and sigma sites with nearly equal affinity.

It has been suggested that antipsychotic activity and extrapyramidal side effects (EPS) may reside in different pathways in the brain (Carlsson 1978). The antipsychotic effect may reside in the limbic structures and the extrapyramidal effects in the striatum. This hypothesis could be tested with PET if the relevant labeled drugs were available.

There is a renewed interest in the atypical neuroleptic clozapine in part because of the minimal ability of this drug and other atypical drugs to produce EPS. One hypothesis for the mode of action suggests that the relative affinity of this drug for the serotonin receptor system in contrast to the affinity for the dopamine receptor system may have a significant role in the ability of this drug to relieve some of the symptoms of psychosis while producing minimal EPS (Matsubara and Meltzer 1989).

The role of other receptor systems in producing EPS is also unclear (Creese 1985). There is some indirect evidence that there is a correlation between the amount of time a neuroleptic is bound to a receptor and the EPS. The longer the drug is bound the greater the EPS.

METHODS FOR THE MEASUREMENT OF RECEPTOR DENSITY WITH PET

Receptor imaging is possible with PET because of the high sensitivity of PET when compared with other imaging modalities. Most of the receptors of interest in schizophrenia exist in nanomolar concentration in the living brain. As a result, it requires a technique that can measure these levels accurately. The PET measurement of the concentration of the radiolabeled drug does not give the information needed to directly make an assessment of the receptor number or affinity. To make these assessments requires the use of a model of the system (Frost 1988). Simpler methods may be used to estimate some of the parameters once these estimates have been shown to be valid by doing a complete kinetic analysis of the system. The application and interpretation of the PET data are subjects of some controversy and the resolution should give insight into the physiological processes involved.

There are two basic methods to determine the distribution of ligands in specific areas of the brain. The first of these is the direct visualization of the ligand bound to the receptor that requires that the ligand of interest be tagged with the radiolabel. The second indirect method is to use a radiolabeled ligand specific for a particular receptor and then try to block the uptake of the receptor with the compound of interest. The first method is certainly preferable if the radiolabeled compound can be synthesized, since this method also allows the regional distribution to be determined and gives evidence of the effects of transport and nonspecific binding.

Direct Visualization

The most straightforward method for determining the in vivo distribution and binding characteristics of a new ligand is to label the ligand with a positron-emitting label. This has been done with a number of compounds (Fowler and Wolf 1982; Kilbourn 1990). The biodistribution can be determined directly from the PET image and can be compared directly with the expected distribution based on animal data and the known affinity of the compound with receptor subtypes. The effects of the lipophilicity of the drug as well as any transport system can be evaluated with the application of the appropriate model to the PET data. The receptor that has been studied most thoroughly is the D_2 receptor.

Blocking Experiments

If the radiolabeled ligand of interest can be synthesized, blocking experiments can be done to determine the type of receptor to which it is bound. Often some information as to the receptor type can be inferred from the literature concerning the in vitro data and from the regional distribution of the radiolabeled compound, but the best method is to block the drug with a receptor-specific ligand whose distribution is known and see how much the uptake in the region of interest is decreased. The difference between the receptor affinity in vitro and the distribution in vivo is often quite striking. The role of transport and metabolism is considerable and cannot be ignored when determining the clinical efficacy of a particular drug.

If the radioligand binds to several types of receptors, as is the case with many of the neuroleptics, it is necessary to block one type of receptor while observing the uptake in another. This type of experiment can also often shed light on the amount of nonspecific binding of the radioligand.

Methods of Evaluation

There are many methods being used by PET groups to try and gain useful quantitative information about the receptor system under study. These are those that are irreversibly bound over the usual course of the PET experiment and those that are reversibly bound over the course of the experiment. The most familiar example of the first type (irreversibly bound) is N-methylspiroperidol labeled with either fluorine-18 (^{18}F-NMS; Arnett et al. 1986) or carbon-11 (^{11}C-NMS; Wagner et al. 1983). This ligand does not reach equilibrium during the course of the experiment. This can be easily determined by plotting the bound-free ratio as a function of time for the compound. The bound-free ratio is determined by dividing the concentration of radioligand in a region of interest by the concentration of radioligand in a region with little or no specific binding of the ligand. If the compound is at equilibrium with the tissue, then this ratio should be a constant. In the case of ^{18}F-NMS, the ratio is still increasing even after 4 hours. Since NMS does not reach equilibrium, the mathematical models that make this assumption cannot be used to determine the parameters of the binding.

There are several methods that have been successfully used to analyze the data from ^{18}F-NMS experiments. The simplest of these is the "ratio index" method, which involves plotting the ratio of an area of specific binding to an area of nonspecific binding over time. In the case of ^{18}F-NMS, this means plotting the striatum value over the cerebellum value versus time. It has been shown that this can be related to the receptor density if the assumption is made that the affinity (K_d) values are constant. This technique has been used to determine the extent of receptor occupancy during treatment with neuroleptics (Smith et al. 1988; Wolkin et al. 1989). This method has the distinct advantage of being very simple to use and not requiring arterial blood sampling.

The next in the order of complexity are the Patlak-Gjedde graphical methods, which use the plasma activity value derived from the arterial blood curve and the incorporation of radioactivity in the striatum (Patlak and Blasberg 1985; Patlak et al. 1983; Wong et al. 1986a, 1986b). The derivation of this model is quite involved and requires several assumptions to be made. This technique has been used by several groups for the analysis of labeled NMS data, and the method has been extended to other compounds that are not receptor binding in nature. In a variation of this method, the plasma curve can be replaced with the cerebellar curve with similar results. A rearrangement of the basic equations used to derive the Patlak-Gjedde methods leads to the incorporation quotient as first described by Patlak (1981). The advantage of this method is that it is the ratio of two large numbers (the activity in the region of interest and the plasma integral to that point in time) that tends to minimize the statistical noise in the image as well as variations in the plasma curve.

The most complex method of modeling that can be used for this type of irreversibly bound agent is the three-compartment four-parameter kinetic model or the four-compartment six-parameter kinetic model (Logan et al. 1987; Wong et al. 1986c). Both of these models require an arterial input function as well as a metabolite analysis of the activity in the blood to be accurate. The debate here is whether one is justified in using six parameters when four parameters fit the data just as well. It can be argued that the use of the six parameters most closely resembles what is occurring in the body, but considering the complexity of the actual physiological processes and the simplifications that have already been made in using the six-parameter model, it may not be significantly worse to use the simpler four-parameter model. This is a direct result of the fact that the data themselves have uncertainties of 5–10% associated with them. The uncertainty in the data arises from the scanning and reconstruction procedure, the blood counting, and the plasma analysis. It is not possible at this time to achieve lower noise levels in PET.

In the case of the reversibly bound compound, things can in principle be simpler. It must be demonstrated that the system is truly at equilibrium (Sedvall et al. 1986). Equilibrium is defined as that point when the rates of the forward and reverse chemical reactions (or association reactions) are equal. In some instances, compounds that appear to be at equilibrium are in reality not. An example is [^{11}C]cocaine in humans. If the bound-free ratio (striatum divided by cerebellum in this case) is plotted versus time, the curve goes through a maximum and then decreases. This suggests that the system was momentarily at equilibrium with respect to influx and efflux, but that the efflux of the compound from the tissue could not keep up with the declining levels of tracer in the bloodstream. Thus, the equilibrium methods of analysis could be used in this case only at the time point where the curve went through a maximum. The Patlak-Gjedde methods using the slope of the line of tissue/plasma versus plasma integral/plasma also cannot be used, since the plot of the function is never linear. The incorporation quotient has been used in this case, since the terms that are dependent on time cancel out of the equations (Fowler et al. 1989a, 1989b).

In general, the method of analysis is fairly specific for a particular radioligand, and a method of analysis must be found that is valid for that particular radioligand. The graphical methods are easy to use and seem to be valid for most irreversibly bound ligands. The full kinetic analysis requires a significant amount of computer time and someone who understands how to manipulate the parameters to obtain the best solution to the equations (Zeeberg et al. 1988a, 1988b).

DOPAMINE RECEPTORS

D2 Receptors

The concept that some forms of schizophrenia are inextricably entwined with the D2 receptor is well accepted. The extremely high correlation between the potency of the neuroleptic drugs and their affinity for the D_2 receptor has been clearly demonstrated. There are many complexities even in our present understanding of the dopamine system that can cause difficulties in the interpretation of the data. The current model of the dopamine receptor system is given in Figure 5-6. The feedback loops of the synthesis-modulating autoreceptor (SMAR) and the release-modulating autoreceptor (RMAR) as well as the catabolic pathways may quickly respond to the presence of dopamine in the synaptic cleft. The speed of this response will affect the level of the dopamine during an experiment and could alter the measured value of the receptor concentration depending on the binding characteristics of the ligand used to measure receptor occupancy.

The flow of dopamine into the synapse is regulated at several points, and the drugs used to maintain the dopamine level in the synaptic cleft may cause an effect by acting at any of these points. The classic neuroleptics such as haloperidol, chlorpromazine, and fluphenazine block the D_2 receptor in the postsynaptic membrane. This causes the

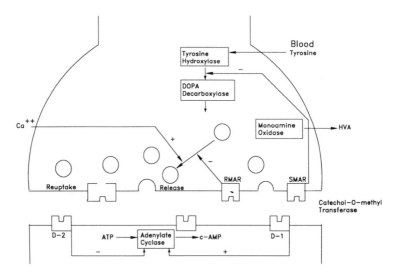

Figure 5-6. Schematic diagram of the dopamine receptor synaptic cleft with the associated feedback loops. HVA = homovanillic acid. RMAR = receptor-modulated autoreceptor. SMAR = synthesis-modulated autoreceptor. A positive symbol (+) indicates that this agent stimulates the next step toward the release of the neurotransmitter, whereas a negative symbol (−) indicates an inhibition of the following step. Rectangular boxes represent enzyme systems in the neuron.

amount of dopamine in the synaptic cleft to increase and blocks the transmission of the signal along the neuron. Drugs such as cocaine or nomifensine that block the reuptake of the dopamine into the presynaptic neuron also increase the levels of dopamine in the synaptic cleft. The difference is that the neuroleptics cause a diminution of the signal being passed through the synapse, whereas cocaine, nomifensine, and similar drugs allow the signal to be passed and increase sensitivity.

PET has been used to assess whether there are changes in the number of D_2 receptors in schizophrenic patients. Previous postmortem studies had demonstrated that some schizophrenic patients had increases in the number of D_2 receptors. The results were confounded by the fact that they were not done in the living human brain and that most of the brains studied were from patients who had a history of previous neuroleptic treatment. The PET studies were able to measure the D_2 receptor density in the brain of living schizophrenic patients who had never received neuroleptic treatment (Farde et al. 1986, 1987a; Wong 1986a). The two studies came to opposite conclusions so that no definitive answer is yet available. It is not clear at this point if the difference lies in the patients chosen or in the technique used to measure the receptor density. A report has recently been written about the various possibilities (Andreasen et al. 1988), but no definite conclusion had been reached at the time of this writing. It seems most likely that the answer lies in the affinity of the two ligands used to determine receptor density. It has been clearly shown in vitro that the affinity of the ligand used toward the D_2 receptor will have an effect on the apparent receptor density as determined with PET (Seeman et al. 1989). If the ligand has a high affinity for the receptor as NMS does, then the receptor concentration as measured by PET will be nearly constant as the concentration of endogenous dopamine is changed. If, on the other hand, the affinity of the ligand is close to that of dopamine, the apparent receptor density will change as dopamine concentration in the synapse is changed, since dopamine will compete effectively with the labeled drug for the available sites.

In interpreting these results, it should be kept in mind that there may be a group of schizophrenic patients with elevated D_2 receptor levels and a group with no D_2 receptor density increase. The work of Seeman et al. (1984) in postmortem brains of schizophrenic patients in which a bimodal distribution of D_2 receptors was observed supports this notion. This distinction may also be of relevance to the responder versus nonresponder categories of schizophrenic patients, i.e., those who respond favorably to neuroleptic treatment as opposed to those who do not respond well to this therapy (Wolkin et al. 1989).

Schizophrenia may represent a heterogeneous disease with sub-categories corresponding to different pathological processes that produce similar behavior patterns (DeLisi et al. 1985b).

D_1 Receptors

D_1 receptors have not until recently been considered as relevant in the etiopathogenesis of schizophrenia. A recent study has shown (Hess et al. 1987) that in postmortem brains the D_1 receptor density was significantly decreased in schizophrenic patients as compared with a control group. This investigation also showed an increase in the D_1 receptor affinity (K_d) in the brains of schizophrenic patients. In addition, the schizophrenic individual showed an increase in the D_2 receptor density (56%). It is at odds with another study that showed no such increase in postmortem brains of schizophrenic patients (Pimoule et al. 1985).

Evidence suggests that there may be a synergistic effect between the D_1 and D_2 receptor systems, and certain dopamine-mediated behaviors are antagonized by combinations of D_1 and D_2 antagonists more effectively than by either one of them alone (Beaulieu 1987; Carlson et al. 1987). The ratio of activity of the D_2 to the D_1 receptor may be important in understanding psychopathology in schizophrenic patients (Clark and White 1987). Preliminary PET studies have been done to map the D_1 receptor distribution in the human brain (Farde et al. 1987a, 1987b). PET studies are underway to characterize the ability of different neuroleptics to block the D_1 versus the D_2 receptors in the human brain and the relationship between their D_1/D_2 blocking ability and their effectiveness (Lundberg et al. 1989).

SIGMA RECEPTORS

The sigma receptor was first identified by the binding of N-allylnormetazocine (NANM) in the brain of rats (Martin et al. 1976). It was clearly different from the PCP receptor that was in large part responsible for its discovery and that is associated with the N-methyl-D-aspartate (NMDA) receptors. A classification system to distinguish the principal differences between the sigma site and the PCP site has been proposed (Quirion et al. 1987). Some of the typical neuroleptic drugs such as haloperidol show strong binding to the sigma sites. In fact, haloperidol has an affinity for sigma receptors at least as strong as its affinity for the D_2 receptor. It has been shown that sigma-selective drugs injected into the brains of rats cause movement disorders that are similar in nature to the side effects caused by the common neuroleptics (Walker et al. 1988). The distribution of sigma sites in postmortem human brain has been determined using ^{3}H-labeled haloperidol (Table 5-1; Weissman et al. 1988).

Role of Sigma Receptors

There has been growing interest in the role of sigma receptors in the course of mental disorders since the identification of these receptors as a class of receptors separate from the opiate receptors. There have been several studies relating the affinity of these receptors with the psychiatric disorder of schizophrenia (Largent et al. 1988; Snyder and Largent 1989). It is known that many of the more effective neuroleptics also bind to the sigma receptor. It has been suggested that screening of new drugs for the treatment of these disorders may be done by determining the affinity of a new drug for the sigma receptor (Manallack et al. 1988).

It is hoped that new drugs that act through different mechanisms from the classic neuroleptics may offer a chance for effective therapy that does not have the commonly associated side effects. One mechanism of action that has been receiving considerable attention is through the sigma receptors. Models using rodent behavior as a test have been made on several drugs, and some promising drugs have been discovered. It may be possible to label these drugs with a positron-emitting compound and thereby determine the distribution and relative receptor occupancy of a new drug. The experience with ^{18}F-labeled haloperidol has shown that receptor affinity is not the only

Table 5-1. Distribution of sigma receptors in the human brain

Brain region	Receptor density (fmole/mg protein)
Cerebellar cortex	130 ± 8
Orbitofrontal cortex	111 ± 18
Nucleus accumbens	110 ± 23
Occipital pole cortex	106 ± 15
Frontal pole cortex	101 ± 5
Superior temporal gyrus	97 ± 4
Somatosensory cortex	86 ± 16
Caudate nucleus	84 ± 17
Hippocampus formation	73 ± 22
Substantia nigra	71 ± 8
Thalamus	58 ± 14
Cervical spinal cord	56 ± 7
Pontine nuclei	45 ± 9

Note. Receptor densities are means ± SD.
Source. Data from Weissman et al. 1988.

factor that needs to be considered when trying to find new drugs that may offer therapeutic benefit.

Examples of Sigma Drugs

Rimcazole shows some efficacy in the treatment of schizophrenia and is essentially inactive at the D_2, S_2, and other receptor sites (Snyder and Largent 1989). This drug is bound with good efficiency to the sigma sites in the brain and may be giving the therapeutic effect through this pathway (Beart et al. 1989).

The distribution of ^{18}F-haloperidol in the human brain shows how the sigma receptors may be bound by this drug (D. J. Schlyer, C. Y. Shiue, J. S. Fowler, et al., 1990, unpublished observations). There can be little doubt that some of either the primary effects of haloperidol or the extrapyramidal side effects of the drug are caused in part by the binding to the sigma receptors. To date it has not been possible to specifically block the sigma receptors with another drug in humans to determine the difference in uptake.

In the area of psychopharmacological research, it has been shown that psychoactive drugs that bind with high affinity to the sigma receptor tend to be more effective in alleviating the "negative symptoms" of schizophrenia such as depression and anxiety in those patients in whom the drugs are effective, whereas psychoactive drugs that have a high affinity for the D_2 sites are more effective in alleviating the "positive symptoms" of schizophrenia.

PET can play a role in the evaluation of these hypotheses by allowing measurement of the in vivo affinity of these psychoactive drugs to the sigma receptor and by determining, in vivo, the possible disruption in the sigma receptors of subgroups of schizophrenic patients. The actual availability of these drugs can be quite different from that predicted on the basis of the in vitro receptor affinity. It is the availability in living humans that is the critical factor in the effectiveness of these drugs.

OTHER RECEPTOR TYPES

Other receptor systems such as the serotonin, gamma-aminobutyric acid (GABA), and the excitatory amino acid NMDA have also been implicated in the etiopathogenesis of schizophrenia (Hanada et al. 1987; Kerwin et al. 1988). One strategy to test the involvement of a given neurotransmitter in schizophrenia has been to correlate the therapeutic efficacy of a neuroleptic with the affinity for a particular type of receptor site. This task is a difficult one in the sense that the known correlation between drug efficacy and D_2 receptors may overshadow other weaker interactions. One such study was carried out with 22 neuroleptics and serotonin, α-adrenergic, and histamine receptors (Peroutka and Snyder 1980). The clinical doses of the neuroleptics used correlated extremely well with the affinity for the D_2 receptor but not at all with the other receptor systems. It may well be that the binding at these other systems has a powerful effect on the extrapyramidal symptoms demonstrated in patients on neuroleptic therapy.

This strategy has also been utilized to characterize the unique therapeutic profile of clozapine, an antipsychotic agent effective for the alleviation of "negative symptoms." In the case of clozapine, its therapeutic efficacy has been related by some to its ability to block serotonin receptors and by others to its ratio of D_1/D_2 receptor blockade (Meltzer et al. 1989). Preliminary work with PET to monitor the distribution and blocking of clozapine in the brain has been achieved with [^{11}C]clozapine (Lundberg et al. 1989). This study showed a widespread distribution in the cortex and subcortical structures. No blocking experiments were done to determine the nature of the binding.

Serotonin

Another strategy has been to measure the concentration of the different receptor types in the brain of diagnosed schizophrenic patients. Postmortem studies have demonstrated decreased serotonin receptors in brains of schizophrenic patients (Bennett et al. 1979). It is known that most of the neuroleptic drugs have some serotonergic component in their binding characteristics (Mumford et al. 1978). Indirect evidence is also provided by studies investigating regions with a high density of serotonergic receptors such as the frontal cortex. These studies appear to show that many patients with schizophrenia manifest clinical symptoms suggestive of prefrontal cortex dysfunction (Weinberger 1988b). There have been several PET studies to determine the metabolic rate in the prefrontal cortex of schizophrenic patients (Buchsbaum et al. 1984; DeLisi et al. 1985a; Farkas et al. 1984; Widen et al. 1981; Wolkin et al. 1985). The reports are conflicting and no clear picture has emerged, but several studies suggest a hypofrontality (Buchsbaum et al. 1984; Wolkin et al. 1985).

NMDA Receptors and Others

Glutamate can be neurotoxic, an effect mediated in part by the NMDA receptor complex. The role of this complex in schizophrenia is currently under investigation with PET using ^{11}C-labeled MK-801 as a PET tracer for the NMDA receptor (Wong et al. 1989). This is an application of PET to confirm in vivo the results obtained in postmortem brains using ^{3}H-labeled MK-801 (Kornhuber et al. 1989a).

The role of the other receptor systems in the etiopathogenesis of schizophrenia and their role in the clinical efficacy and the extrapyramidal side effects of the neuroleptics is now beginning to be explored with PET. The correlation between drug response and receptor availability is an area where PET can play an active role in the future.

IN VIVO DISTRIBUTION OF NEUROLEPTICS

There have been several studies done with PET where the in vivo distribution of D_2 receptors using labeled neuroleptics or analogue drugs have been carried out. The first of these with a highly selective agent was with ^{11}C-NMS (Wagner et al. 1983). The distribution observed was that expected of a D_2 antagonist. A similar study was carried out with ^{18}F-NMS that showed an identical distribution as would be expected (Arnett et al. 1986). The distribution of ^{18}F-NMS is shown in Figure 5-7. The high uptake in the basal ganglia and low

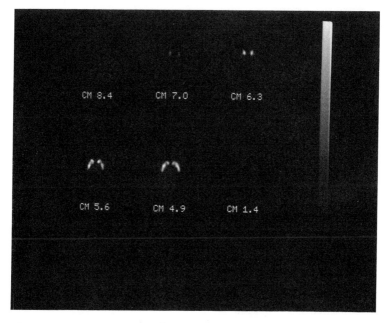

Figure 5-7. Distribution of ^{18}F-labeled *N*-methylspiroperidol in the human brain (Arnett et al. 1986).

uptake in the rest of the brain is exactly the distribution of D2 sites in the brain. The correlation between the receptor density as measured in vitro and the uptake in the various regions of the brain is shown in Figure 5-8. The linear relationship demonstrates that the NMS is binding nearly exclusively to D2 receptors at 3 hours postinjection.

The fact that haloperidol blocks the uptake of ^{18}F-NMS in the striatum suggests that this drug must be binding to the D2 receptor. When ^{18}F-haloperidol was prepared and injected into human subjects, it was clear that the distribution did not reflect the distribution of D2 receptors in the same way that ^{18}F-NMS did. A comparison of the distribution of ^{18}F-haloperidol to that of ^{18}F-NMS is shown in Figure 5-9. The distribution of the haloperidol is widespread and probably reflects uptake at a number of receptor subtypes, especially the sigma receptor, as well as nonspecific binding. There is not a linear correlation between the measured in vitro receptor densities and the uptake in the various regions of the brain.

The distribution of ^{11}C-labeled raclopride has also been determined in humans (Farde et al. 1985, 1987b). The distribution is very

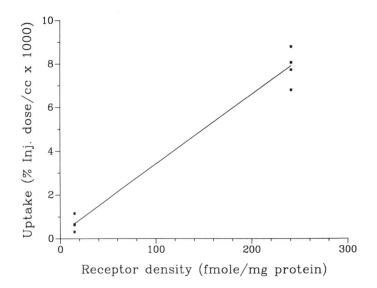

Figure 5-8. Correlation between the in vitro D2 receptor density of different regions of the brain with the observed uptake of N-methylspiroperidol in that region. Uptake is taken from Arnett et al. 1986 and receptor density is taken from Luabeya et al. 1984.

similar to that for ^{18}F-NMS at longer times. The drug washes out of the striatum much more quickly than the ^{18}F-NMS due to the lower affinity of raclopride for the D_2 receptor. This lower affinity has some advantages and disadvantages when used to measure the binding potential of the D_2 receptor. The lower affinity means that ^{11}C-raclopride will be in competition with the dopamine present in the synapse. Thus, the measured level of receptors can be influenced by differences in the levels of endogenous dopamine. This effect will cause problems when trying to measure absolute receptor densities unless it can be demonstrated that the dopamine levels in the inter-synaptic cleft are so small that they do not compete effectively. This competition may be an advantage if a study wishes to observe effects on the levels of dopamine when other drugs are given.

The distribution and binding have also been studied with PET for

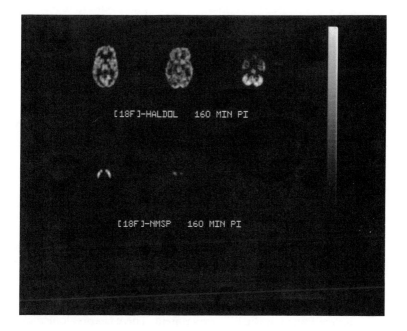

Figure 5-9. Comparison of the distribution of ^{18}F-labeled *N*-methylspi-roperidol (^{18}F-NMSP) with the distribution of ^{18}F-labeled haloperidol in the human brain. Distribution of the haloperidol does not follow the D_2 receptor distribution (D.J. Schlyer, C.Y. Shiue, J.S. Fowler, et al., 1990, unpublished observations).

chlorpromazine and clozapine (Comar et al. 1979; Lundberg et al. 1989). In the case of chlorpromazine, its metabolism makes interpretation of the PET data difficult, since the metabolites also cross the blood-brain barrier and are incorporated into the tissue.

DRUG DESIGN AND EXTRAPYRAMIDAL SIDE EFFECTS

One of the most serious problems associated with neuroleptic therapy is that nearly all these drugs cause some EPS. The causes of these effects are not known with certainty, but they are likely related to the binding potential of the neuroleptic drugs with the neurotransmitter receptor systems. It has been shown that the sedative effects of the neuroleptics correlate well with the α-adrenergic binding potential and that the motor dysfunctions are associated with binding at the cholinergic receptors.

One way PET can make a great contribution to the field of neuropharmacology is to determine the distribution of the drugs and correlate this distribution with the binding potential at a series of different sites in vivo. This distribution can be quite different from the in vitro affinity of the drug for the receptors, since the distribution of these lipophilic drugs is often not directly related to the regional receptor density and affinity of the drug for the receptor. Once the correlation between the EPS and the receptor occupancy has been determined, new drugs can be designed to maximize the therapeutic effect while minimizing the EPS.

CONCLUSIONS: FUTURE OF PET IN MENTAL DISORDERS

The real contributions that PET can make to the field of psychiatry are in understanding the physiological basis for the disease and in the design and evaluation of new therapeutic agents. In addition, the correlation of drug dosage with receptor occupancy can provide objective information on the therapeutic dosage levels. The observed binding profile of the drug when compared with the clinical effect can yield understanding of the basis of action. New drugs can be developed by altering their design until they give desired binding profiles as determined by the PET experiment. These factors alone make PET very powerful in both the understanding of the disease and the methods of treatment.

REFERENCES

Andreasen NC, Carson RC, Diksic M, et al: Proceedings of a workshop on schizophrenia, PET, and dopamine D2 receptors in the human neostriatum. Schizophr Bull 14:471–484, 1988

Arnett CD, Wolf AP, Shiue C-Y, et al: Improved delineation of human dopamine receptors using [^{18}F]- *N*-methylspiroperidol and PET. J Nucl Med 27:1878–1882, 1986

Beart PM, O'Shea RD, Manallack DT: Regulation of σ-receptors: high- and low-affinity agonist states, GTP shifts, and up-regulation by rimcazole and 1,3-di(2-tolyl)guanidine. J Neurochem 53:779–788, 1989

Beaulieu M: Clinical importance of D-1 and D-2 receptors. Can J Neurol Sci 14:402–406, 1987

Bennett JP, Enna SJ, Bylund DB, et al: Neurotransmitter receptors in frontal cortex of schizophrenics. Arch Gen Psychiatry 36:927–934, 1979

Buchsbaum MS, DeLisi LE, Holcomb HH, et al: Anteroposterior gradients in cerebral glucose use in schizophrenia and affective disorders. Arch Gen Psychiatry 41:1159–1166, 1984

Cambon H, Baron JC, Boulenger JP, et al: In vivo assay for neuroleptic receptor binding in the striatum. Br J Psychiatry 151:824–830, 1987

Carlson JH, Bergstrom DA, Walters JR: Stimulation of both D1 and D2 dopamine receptors appears necessary for the full expression of postsynaptic effects of dopamine antagonists: a neurophysiological study. Brain Res 400:205–216, 1987

Carlsson A: Antipsychotic drugs, neurotransmitters, and schizophrenia. Am J Psychiatry 135:164–173, 1978

Clark D, White FJ: Review: D1 dopamine receptor—the search for a function: a critical evaluation of the D1/D2 dopamine receptor classification and its functional implications. Synapse 1:347–388, 1987

Closse A, Frick W, Dravid A, et al: Classification of drugs according to receptor binding profiles. Arch Pharmacol 327:95–101, 1984

Comar D, Zaritian E, Verhas M, et al: Brain distribution and kinetics of ^{11}C-chlorpromazine in schizophrenia: positron emission tomography. Psychiatry Res 1:23–29, 1979

Creese I: Receptor binding as a primary drug screen, in Neurotransmitter Receptor Binding, 2nd Edition. Edited by Yamamura HI. New York, Raven, 1985, pp 189–233

Crow TJ: Left brain, retrotransposons, and schizophrenia. Br Med J 293:3–4, 1986

Delay J, Deniker P, Harl J-M: Traitement des états d'excitation et d'agitation par une méthode médicamenteuse dérivée de l'hibernothérapie. Ann Med Psychol 110:267–273, 1952

DeLisi LE, Buchsbaum MS, Holcomb HH: Clinical correlates of decreased anteroposterior metabolic gradients in positron emission tomography (PET) of schizophrenic patients. Am J Psychiatry 142:78–81, 1985a

DeLisi LE, Goldin LR, Gershon ES, et al: Subgroups in schizophrenia. Lancet 1502, 1985b

Farde L, Ehrin E, Eriksson L, et al: Substituted benzamides as ligands for visualization of dopamine receptor binding in the human brain by positron emission tomography. Proc Natl Acad Sci USA 82:3863–3867, 1985

Farde L, Hall H, Ehrin E, et al: Quantitative analysis of D2 dopamine receptor binding in the living human brain by PET. Science 231: 258–261, 1986

Farde L, Wiesel FA, Hall H, et al: No D_2 receptor increase in PET study of schizophrenia (letter). Arch Gen Psychiatry 44:671, 1987a

Farde L, Halldin C, Stone-Elander S, et al: PET analysis of human dopamine receptor subtypes using ^{11}C-SCH 23390 and ^{11}C-raclopride. Psychopharmacology 92:278–284, 1987b

Farkas T, Wolf AP, Jaeger J, et al: Regional glucose metabolism in chronic schizophrenia. Arch Gen Psychiatry 41:293–300, 1984

Fowler JS, Wolf AP: The Synthesis of Carbon-11, Fluorine-18, and Nitrogen-13 Labeled Radiotracers for Biomedical Applications (Nuclear Science Series NAS-NS-3201). Springfield, VA, National Academy of Science, 1982

Fowler JS, Volkow ND, Wolf AP, et al: [11]C]Cocaine binding in human and baboon brain (abstract). J Nucl Med 5:761, 1989a

Fowler JS, Volkow ND, Wolf AP, et al: [11]C]Cocaine binding in human and baboon brain. Synapse 4:371–377, 1989b

Frost JJ: Receptor localization and quantification with PET. Radiology 169:273–274, 1988

Hanada M, Mita T, Nishino N, et al: [3]H]Muscimol binding sites increased in autopsied brains of chronic schizophrenics. Life Sci 40:259–266, 1987

Hess EJ, Bracha HS, Kleinman JE, et al: Dopamine receptor subtype imbalance in schizophrenia. Life Sci 40:1487–1497, 1987

Kerwin RW, Patel S, Meldrum BS, et al: Asymmetrical loss of glutamate receptor subtype in left hippocampus in schizophrenia. Lancet 1:583, 1988

Kilbourn MR: Fluorine-18 Labelling of Radiopharmaceuticals (National Research Council Nuclear Science Series NAS-NS-3203). Washington, DC, National Academy Press, 1990

Kornhuber J, Reiderer P, Reynolds GP, et al: 3H-Spiperone binding sites in post-mortem brains from schizophrenic patients: relationship to neuroleptic drug treatment, abnormal movements, and positive symptoms. J Neural Transm 75:1–10, 1989b

Largent BL, Wikstrom H, Snowman AM, et al: Novel antipsychotic drugs share high affinity for σ receptors. Eur J Pharmacol 155:345–347, 1988

Logan J, Wolf AP, Shiue CY, et al: Kinetic modeling of receptor-ligand binding applied to positron emission tomographic studies with neuroleptic tracers. J Neurochem 48:73–83, 1987

Luabeya MK, Maloteaux JM, Laduron PM: Regional and cortical laminar distributions of serotonin S_2, benzodiazepine, muscarinic, and dopamine D_2 receptors in human brain. J Neurochem 43:1068–1071, 1984

Lundberg T, Lindstroem LH, Harvig P, et al: Striatal and frontal cortex binding of ^{11}C-labelled clozapine visualized by positron emission tomography (PET) in drug-free schizophrenics and healthy volunteers. Psychopharmacology 99:8–12, 1989

Manallack DT, Wong MG, Cost M, et al: Receptor site topographies for phencyclidine-like and σ drugs: predictions from quantitative conformational, electrostatic potential, and radioreceptor analyses. Mol Pharmacol 34:863–879, 1988

Martin WR, Eades CG, Thompson JA, et al: The effects of morphine- and nalorphine-like drugs in the nondependent and morphine-dependent chronic spinal dog. J Pharmacol Exp Ther 197:517–532, 1976

Matsubara S, Meltzer HY: Effect of typical and atypical antipsychotic drugs on 5-HT$_2$ receptor density in rat cerebral cortex. Life Sci 45:1397–1406, 1989

Meltzer HY, Matsubara S, Lee JC: Classification of typical and atypical antipsychotic drugs on the basis of dopamine D-1, D-2 and serotonin pKi values. J Pharmacol Exp Ther 251:238–246, 1989

Mumford L, Teixeira AR, Kumar R: Serotonergic component of neuroleptic receptors. Nature 272:168, 1978

Patlak CS: Derivation of the equations for the steady-state reaction velocity of a substance based on the use of a second substance. J Cereb Blood Flow Metab 1:129–131, 1981

Patlak CS, Blasberg RG: Graphical evaluation of blood-to-brain transfer constants from multiple-time uptake data: generalizations. J Cereb Blood Flow Metab 5:584–590, 1985

Patlak CS, Blasberg RG, Fenestermacher JD: Graphical evaluation of blood-to-brain transfer constants from multiple-time update data. J Cereb Blood Flow Metab 3:1–7, 1983

Peroutka SJ, Snyder SH: Relationship of neuroleptic drug effects in brain dopamine, serotonin, α-adrenergic, and histamine receptors to clinical potency. Am J Psychiatry 137:1518–1522, 1980

Pimoule C, Schoemaker H, Reynolds GP, et al: [^{3}H]SCH 23390 labeled D_1 dopamine receptors are unchanged in schizophrenia and Parkinson's disease. Eur J Pharmacol 114:235–237, 1985

Quirion R, Chicheportiche R, Contreras PC, et al: Classification and nomenclature of phencyclidine and sigma receptor sites. Topics in Neurosciences 10:443, 1987

Sedvall G, Farde L, Persson A, et al: Imaging of neurotransmitter receptors in the living human brain. Arch Gen Psychiatry 43:995–1005, 1986

Seeman P: Brain dopamine receptors. Pharmacol Rev 32:229–313, 1981

Seeman P: Dopamine receptors and the dopamine hypothesis of schizophrenia. Synapse 1:133–152, 1987

Seeman P, Ulpian C, Bergeron C, et al: Bimodal distribution of dopamine densities in brains of schizophrenics. Science 225:728–731, 1984

Seeman P, Guan HC, Niznik HB: Endogenous dopamine lowers the dopamine D_2 receptor density as measured by [^{3}H]raclopride: implications for positron emission tomography of the human brain. Synapse 3:96–97, 1989

Smith M, Wolf AP, Brodie JF, et al: Serial [^{18}F] N-methylspiroperidol PET studies to measure changes in antipsychotic drug D-2 receptor occupancy in schizophrenic patients. Biol Psychiatry 23:653–663, 1988

Snyder SH, Largent BL: Receptor mechanisms in antipsychotic drug action: focus on sigma receptors. J Neuropsychiatry 1:7–15, 1989

Trimble MR: The neurology of schizophrenia. Br Med Bull 43:587–598, 1987

Vinick FJ, Heym JH: Antipsychotic agents. Annual Reports in Medicinal Chemistry 22:5–10, 1987

Wagner HN, Burns HD, Dannals RF, et al: Imaging dopamine receptors in the human brain by positron tomography. Science 221:1264–1266, 1983

Walker JM, Matsumoto RR, Bowen WD: Evidence for a role of haloperidol-sensitive σ-'opiate' receptors in the motor effects of antipsychotic drugs. Neurology 38:961–965, 1988

Weinberger DR: Premorbid neuropathology in schizophrenia (letter). Lancet 2:445, 1988a

Weinberger DR: Schizophrenia and the frontal lobe. Topics in Neurosciences 11:367, 1988b

Weissman AD, Su TP, Hedreen JC, et al: Sigma receptors in post-mortem human brains. J Pharmacol Exp Ther 247:29–33, 1988

Widen L, Bergstrom M, Blomqvist G, et al: Glucose metabolism in patients with schizophrenia: emission computed tomography measurements with 11-C-glucose. J Cereb Blood Flow Metab 1 (suppl 1):S455–S456, 1981

Wolkin A, Jaeger J, Brodie JD, et al: Persistence of cerebral metabolic abnormalities in chronic schizophrenia as determined by positron emission tomography. Am J Psychiatry 142:564–571, 1985

Wolkin A, Barouche F, Wolf AP, et al: Dopamine blockade and clinical response: evidence for two biological subgroups of schizophrenia. Am J Psychiatry 146:905–908, 1989

Wong DF, Wagner HN, Tune LE, et al: Positron emission tomography reveals elevated D_2 dopamine receptors in drug-naive schizophrenics. Science 234:1558–1563, 1986a

Wong DF, Gjedde A, Wagner HN: Quantification of neuroreceptors in the living human brain, I: irreversible binding of ligands. J Cereb Blood Flow Metab 6:137–146, 1986b

Wong DF, Gjedde A, Wagner HN, et al: Quantification of neuroreceptors in the living human brain, II: inhibition studies of receptor density and affinity. J Cereb Blood Flow Metab 6:147–153, 1986c

Wong DF, Burns HD, Solomon HF, et al: Imaging of NMDA receptor sites with (+)-[C-11]-8-methoxy-MK-801 in vivo by PET (abstract). J Nucl Med 30:741, 1989

Zeeberg BR, Gibson RE, Reba RC: Elevated D_2 dopamine receptors in drug-naive schizophrenics. Science 239:789, 1988a

Zeeberg BR, Gibson RE, Reba RC: Accuracy of in vivo neuroreceptor quantification by PET and review of steady-state, transient, double injection, and equilibrium models. IEEE Transactions in Medical Imaging 6 3:244–249, 1988b

Chapter 6

Quantification of Human Neuroreceptors in Neuropsychiatric Disorders With Positron-Emission Tomography

Dean F. Wong, M.D., and L. Trevor Young, M.D.

Neuroreceptors and neurotransmitter systems in the human brain are presently under investigation with positron-emission tomography (PET) at a number of centers. Since in vivo quantification of human neuroreceptors has only been accomplished in the last decade, such techniques continue to be modified and validated. One of the earliest studies in which PET was used to quantify neuroreceptors suggested a decline in the density of central D_2 neuroreceptors with age (Wong et al. 1984). Although there has been a steady improvement in imaging methods, controversy has surrounded many of the findings obtained with these techniques. Nonetheless, potential findings in neuropsychiatric illnesses stimulate future investigation and may provide real insight into the pathophysiology of these disorders.

Abnormalities in neuroreceptor binding have been demonstrated in a number of neuropsychiatric disorders including schizophrenia (Farde et al. 1987; Wong et al. 1986c), temporal lobe epilepsy (Frost

Special acknowledgments go to clinical collaborators Drs. L.E. Tune, G.D. Pearlson, and C. Ross, who were responsible for the recruitment and characterization of patients in addition to sharing in hypothesis testing in schizophrenic and bipolar patients; to Drs. R.F. Dannals, H. Ravert, and A. Wilson, who were responsible for radioligand production and development; to Drs. M. Kuhar and H.N. Wagner, Jr., for helpful discussions; to Dr. D. Young for HPLC method development; to Drs. A. Gjedde, P.D. Wilson, and R.D. Parker for modeling and statistical considerations; and to Dr. S. Resnick for comments on the manuscript. Thanks go to D. Burkhardt, E. Balcavage, E. Minkin, and B. Chan for technical assistance. This work was supported in part by NIMH Contract RO1-MH-42821 (D.F.W.) and the Medical Research Council of Canada (L.T.Y.).

et al. 1988), poststroke depression (Mayberg et al. 1988), bipolar affective disorder (Wong et al. 1988), and Tourette's syndrome (Wong et al. 1988). To illustrate recent PET techniques developed to quantify neuroreceptors in neuropsychiatric disorders, we will review some of the recent PET studies that have examined human D_2 receptors and then focus on more sophisticated methods that allow estimation of dopamine receptor density (B_{max}). While results obtained with these methods are of interest on their own, they also serve to illustrate important methodological and clinical issues that need to be addressed in the design and interpretation of PET neuroreceptor studies in neuropsychiatric disorders.

D_2 NEURORECEPTOR IMAGING

Historical Perspective

A number of research centers have examined dopamine neuroreceptors with PET since our study in 1983 that demonstrated specific binding to neuroreceptors in living human brain for the first time (Wagner et al. 1983). Since the dopamine neurotransmitter system has been implicated in the etiology of schizophrenia and other major psychiatric disorders with prominent psychotic symptoms, a great deal of effort has been focused on the development of specific PET techniques to quantify human dopamine receptors. Numerous lines of evidence link the dopaminergic neurotransmitter system to schizophrenia. For instance, the antipsychotic action of neuroleptic drugs is correlated with the blockade of D_2 receptors (Creese et al. 1976; Seeman et al. 1976). Increased numbers of D_2 receptors have been detected in postmortem studies of the brains of schizophrenic patients (Lee et al. 1978; Owen et al. 1978). A major issue complicating such postmortem findings has been the history of neuroleptic treatment (Burt et al. 1977; Creese et al. 1977; Mackay et al. 1982). Such strong evidence and specific limitations of in vitro laboratory methods point out the importance of examining dopamine neuroreceptors in living human brains; this can be accomplished with PET.

These basic scientific and clinical findings stimulated a number of attempts to measure D_2 receptors in human brains with PET. Most studies have employed positron-labeled neuroleptic derivatives and then examined simple ratios of specific to nonspecific binding of these ligands (in the case of D_2 receptors, this is usually determined by the caudate to cerebellar ratio). One of the earliest studies was accomplished with ^{11}C-labeled chlorpromazine (Comar et al. 1979); however, specific binding was not clearly visualized. Our center focused on a butyrophenone, ^{11}C-labeled N-methylspiperone (^{11}C-NMSP), and in 1983 it clearly demonstrated specific binding to neuroreceptors in human brains with PET (Wagner et al. 1983). The following year, using ratio methods, we found a fall in dopamine receptors with age in both male and female subjects with the same ligand. Other approaches include the use of ^{18}F-labeled haloperidol, which was limited to nonhuman studies until recently (Logan et al. 1989; Tewson et al. 1980; Welch et al. 1983). Butyrophenone derivatives that have also been studied include benperidol (Arnett et al. 1985) and alkyl derivatives of spiperone (Barrio et al. 1986; Smith et al. 1986; Welch et al. 1986). Several centers have employed bromospiperone as a D_2 receptor ligand in drug-treated schizophrenic patients, with PET (Maziere et al. 1985) and planar imaging (Crawley et al. 1986). Both of these studies with bromospiperone found elevated caudate-to-cerebellar ratios of specific binding in schizophrenic subjects.

Given the limitations of PET techniques that rely on simple specific-to-nonspecific binding ratios, a number of groups, including Perlmutter et al. (1986) and Huang et al. (1986), began to develop kinetic models to extend this ratio methodology. These investigators found elevated forward rate binding constants (K_3) in methylphenyltetrahydropyridine (MPTP) Parkinson's disease patients and in baboons in the acute phase of MPTP intoxication (Perlmutter et al. 1987). Another approach to modeling of receptor binding kinetics was developed by Logan et al. (1989), in which two PET scans with high and low specific activity D_2 radioligands are performed. The next step in this effort to image dopamine receptors was the development of methods to estimate D_2 receptor B_{max}. These studies will be considered next.

Newer PET Techniques That Estimate Receptor B_{max}

In 1986, we reported a kinetic model to estimate receptor B_{max} in living human brains (Wong et al. 1986a). Concurrently, Farde et al. (1986) developed a different approach to measure D_2 receptor B_{max} that involves quasi-equilibrium measurement with high and low specific activity scans. To date these are the principal methods that have been developed to measure D_2 receptor B_{max} in brains with PET. Both methods involve at least two scans and a model that is employed to determine these binding parameters. The PET group at Brookhaven National Laboratory has also developed methods to quantify dopamine receptors, but these methods have not been applied to large clinical populations. Both of these methods will be described in more detail later.

With our more sophisticated method requiring two PET scans to determine B_{max}, we showed an approximately twofold elevation in D_2

B_{max} in 10 drug-naive schizophrenic subjects and 5 drug-free schizophrenic patients as compared with 11 normal control subjects (Figure 6-1) using the ligand ^{11}C-NMSP (Wong et al. 1986d). We continue to find elevated receptor density in our sample, which has since been expanded to 20 drug-naive schizophrenic patients (Tune et al. 1989; Wong et al. 1989a, 1989b). Using PET with the radioligand ^{11}C-labeled raclopride, Farde et al. (1987) from the Karolinska Institute failed to demonstrate significant differences in D_2 receptor density or affinity between 15 drug-naive schizophrenic patients and normal control subjects. It has become clear that there are many factors that might contribute to such markedly different findings with these two PET methods to measure D_2 receptor B_{max}. These divergent results from two different centers will serve as an example to illustrate some important methodological and clinical issues regarding PET neuroreceptor imaging in living human brains.

We will also describe our recent work in patients with bipolar affective disorder, as these findings illustrate how collaborative evidence from another neuropsychiatric disorder can bear on the interpretation of PET findings in schizophrenia. The discussion will conclude by addressing several clinical questions that need to be examined to understand the place of PET in psychiatric clinical research.

METHODOLOGICAL ISSUES

Patient and Control Populations

Perhaps due to the complex technology associated with PET scanning, an important issue may not be adequately addressed: characteristics of patient and control populations. Diagnostic criteria and clinical characteristics of patients are fundamental in designing and interpreting clinical investigations, particularly in psychiatry, which has few disease-specific markers or definitive diagnostic tests. As clinical findings vary in the acute and chronic stages of this disorder, neurochemical findings in schizophrenia may be more prominent at later stages of illness rather than at the onset of symptoms. Such a situation would be consistent with computed tomography (CT) scan abnormalities that were found to be more apparent in chronic versus acute schizophrenia (Luchins 1982). As noted above, two PET studies of D_2 receptor findings had different results. Patients from the study from Johns Hopkins University, which found D_2 receptor changes in these patients, were older (mean age 31 ± 4 years, $n = 10$) and had been ill for a longer time (4.7 years), compared with patients in the Swedish study who had negative results (mean age

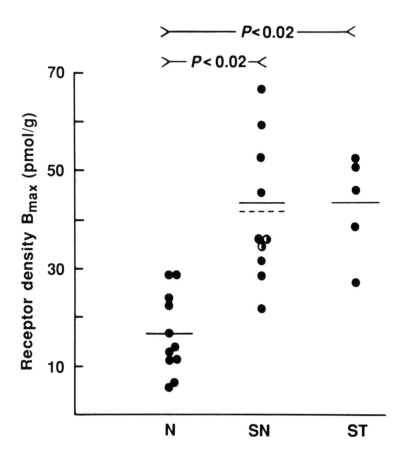

Figure 6-1. D_2 receptor density (B_{max}) in the caudate nucleus in normal volunteers (N) and drug-naive (SN) and drug-treated (ST) schizophrenic patients. *Solid horizontal lines* are the mean values in each group. For the drug-naive group this line is the value for the 8 subjects who had only a single 7.5-mg dose of haloperidol before their second PET scan (43.3 ± 5.7 [SE] pmol/g). *Dotted line* below it is the mean of all 10 subjects, including the 2 who received more than a single dose of haloperidol before their second PET scan. The average receptor density of this group was 41.7 ± 4.6 pmol/g. Mean receptor densities for the normal volunteers and the drug-treated group were 16.6 ± 2.5 and 43.3 ± 4.7 pmol/g, respectively. There was a significant difference (*t* test with Bonferroni correction for multiple inference) between either the 8 or 10 drug-naive or the drug-treated schizophrenic patients and the normal subjects. (Reprinted with permission from Wong et al. 1986d.)

24 ± 4 years, $n = 15$; mean duration of illness 1.9 years). If D_2 receptor changes occur only at a later stage of illness, such clinical issues may be relevant. The duration of illness, time of scanning relative to the first episode, presence or absence of psychotic features, premorbid personality traits, and predominant positive or negative symptoms are just some examples of potentially relevant factors that may be important in interpreting PET neuroreceptor imaging in schizophrenia. In general, it is important to consider all relevant issues related to typical clinical presentations of a specific neuropsychiatric disorder in the design and interpretation of PET studies.

In addition to clinical issues in patient groups, attention must be directed toward the selection of appropriate control groups. Matching on the basis of age and sex is extremely important in the case of D_2 receptor imaging, in which sex differences affect the pattern of the decrease in density with age (Wong et al. 1984). Moreover, socioeconomic status and level of education also need to be considered. In practice, it is difficult to recruit subject groups matched on these variables for such complex procedures as PET neuroreceptor studies. Since an essential feature of schizophrenia is the presence of impairment in social functioning (DSM-III-R, American Psychiatric Association 1987), matching on patient's socioeconomic status and level of education may not be appropriate. In general, patient variables that may confound experimental design need to be considered and subject groups matched on such variables.

Radioligand Pharmacology

Important initial considerations in choosing a PET strategy to quantify a neuroreceptor in vivo in human brains include pharmacologic parameters of the proposed radioligand, such as the kinetics and affinity of binding, selectivity, and specificity. In general, PET radioligands can be divided into two types—those that reach a quasi-equilibrium during the PET scan and those that do not. The first type of ligand—for example, raclopride—is rapidly reversible and displays considerable dissociation during the time interval of the PET scan. In the latter group, nonequilibrating ligands, like NMSP, can be considered to bind "irreversibly" because of minimal dissociation from brain regions during the time frame of the PET scan, which is based on the short half-life of typical radioisotopes (^{11}C, $t_{1/2} = 20$ minutes; ^{18}F, $t_{1/2} = 110$ minutes). Consideration of the reversibility of binding of a particular PET radioligand is one of the most important factors in the development of models to quantify neuroreceptors.

The affinity of a PET radioligand for neuroreceptors of interest is also extremely important. In most cases, in vitro estimates of such binding parameters obtained in animals or postmortem human brains are valuable in choosing a ligand. Differences in the affinity of a ligand for the D_2 receptor are relevant to PET D_2 receptor measurements in schizophrenia. For example, [^{11}C]NMSP used by the Johns Hopkins group has about a 5- to 10-fold higher affinity than that of the published values for ^{11}C-raclopride or ^{3}H-labeled raclopride (Kohler et al. 1985; Lyon et al. 1986). Lower-affinity reversible ligands suggest greater susceptibility to competition from endogenous neurotransmitters. Seeman et al. (1989) found in animal studies reduction in apparent B_{max} in the presence of 100 nM dopamine with ^{3}H-raclopride but not with ^{3}H-labeled NMSP (Figure 6-2). They suggest that this is an important factor that might explain the discrepancies between the Johns Hopkins and Swedish findings, as intrasynaptic dopamine levels may interfere with B_{max} estimates obtained with raclopride. Furthermore, we have recently found that amphetamine (10 mg/kg iv) administered to mice prior to injection reduces the striatal to cerebellar ratios of both ^{3}H-NMSP and ^{3}H-raclopride binding at 30 minutes by approximately 30%, but at 2 hours postinjection such decreases only occur with raclopride binding.

High-affinity ligands that do not reach equilibrium may also be subject to complex receptor ligand interactions. Chugani et al. (1988) suggested that the ^{3}H-labeled spiperone receptor complex was internalized into intracytoplasmic vesicles, in addition to remaining at the synaptic membrane. Such a mechanism, if confirmed, would increase our understanding of the functional and dynamic nature of these receptors being measured by some PET ligands (Figure 6-3).

Modeling Issues

As mentioned earlier in the section on ligand pharmacology, modeling approaches with NMSP, which binds irreversibly, and raclopride, which binds reversibly, are distinctly different. In general, there are two types of models in PET receptor studies—dynamic nonequilibrium and equilibrium—that have been used with the radioligands NMSP and raclopride, respectively.

The Johns Hopkins study used a dynamic model in which two PET scans with ^{11}C-NMSP were performed, unblocked and blocked (haloperidol 7.5 mg po 4 hours before scan) in each subject (Figure 6-4). The B_{max} estimates are derived from the brain haloperidol concentration divided by the difference in the reciprocal of blocked and unblocked rate constants (Wong et al. 1986a). The first type of model, dynamic nonequilibrium, requires the appropriate input function analysis of blood radioactivity, which, in some cases, is crucial to demonstrate differences in patient groups. For example, the initial use

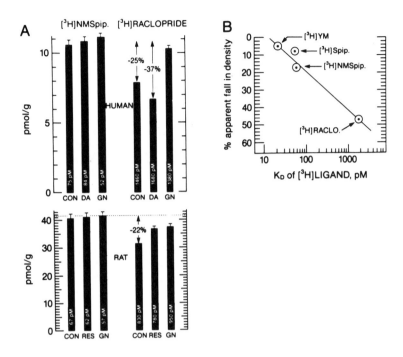

Figure 6-2. *A,* Bars indicate that the D_2 receptor densities, when using ³H-labeled methylspiperone ([³H]NMSpip), were unaffected by exogenous dopamine (DA, 100 nM), by 100 μM guanylimidodiphosphate (GN), or by reserpine (RES, 3 mg/kg ip, 24 hours before death). The D_2 receptor densities when using ³H-labeled raclopride were lower than those obtained when using [³H]NMSpip. For the controls it was reduced 22–25%, and in the presence of 100 nM dopamine the apparent reduction in B_{max} was 37%. Pretreatment of the rats with reserpine prevented the apparent reduction in B_{max} seen in the presence of 100 nM dopamine. Human data are for the same human caudate nucleus (brain T 181) done three times and data averaged. Error bars indicate SE rat data for $N = 4$. Centrifugation method was used throughout (Seeman et al. 1987). The mean K_D value (SE was ± 8%) is shown at the bottom of each bar. CON indicates control values. *B,* Ordinate indicates the apparent fall (in percentage of control) in the density of binding sites for each of four [³H]neuroleptic ligands (YM = YM-09151-2; Spip. = spiperone; Raclo. = raclopride) on the addition of 2,000 nM exogenous dopamine (in 0.1% ascorbic acid in buffered medium, pH 7.4). The K_D of each [³H]ligand was obtained by saturation analysis on human brain striata. Centrifugation method was used. (Reprinted with permission from Seeman et al. 1989.)

PRESYNAPTIC   **POSTSYNAPTIC**

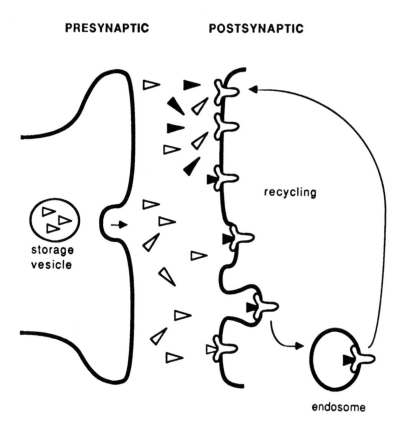

Figure 6-3. Schematic representation of a striatal synaptic junction illustrating some of the complexities associated with PET radioligands binding to D_2 receptors. *Clear triangles* represent endogenous dopamine released from the presynaptic vesicles. *Dark triangles* represent the radiolabeled ligand that is imaged with PET. Two potential pharmacologic parameters that influence PET radioligand binding are shown: competition for binding with endogenous dopamine and internalization of the radioligand–surface receptor complex into the postsynaptic nerve terminal. In the first case, high levels of this endogenous dopamine could compete with their lower-affinity ligand, e.g., [^{11}C]raclopride. In the latter case, internalization of the radioligand–surface receptor complex suggests that PET imaging may reflect functional turnover of surface receptors. Although Chugani et al. (1988) suggested that spiperone may be internalized, this has not yet been replicated by other groups.

of tissue ratios of caudate to cerebellum binding, traditionally used as a measure of specific to nonspecific binding in rodent in vivo studies (Kuhar et al. 1978), failed to demonstrate differences in several diseases, such as Tourette's disorder, schizophrenia, and bipolar disorder (Wong et al. 1985). This is probably due to confounding blood-flow changes that are not taken into consideration by simple tissue ratios but are accounted for by kinetic models (Mintun et al. 1984; Wong et al. 1986a). This potential problem of flow limitation has occurred with a number of ligands under development. Kinetic modeling procedures attempt to distinguish receptor binding components of interest to allow separate estimation of density (B_{max}) and affinity (K_d). In some cases, a "steady-state condition" may be reached between some of the compartments, for instance, nonspecific binding and unmetabolized radioligand in the case of ^{11}C-NMSP for D_2 receptor quantification (Wong et al. 1986a, 1986b). Such conditions can also be used in the model calculations to estimate factors such as the labeled metabolites or partition coefficient for ^{11}C-NMSP. Indeed, analogous steady-state conditions are assumed in the Sokoloff-Phelps-Huang glucose metabolism model (Huang et al. 1980; Sokoloff et al. 1977).

On the other hand, in an equilibrium model (actually, quasi-equilibrium is reached after a bolus injection, since equilibrium requires a constant infusion), the use of simple tissue ratios in a Scatchard-type

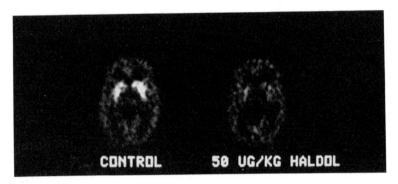

Figure 6-4. Appearance of a typical [11C]N-methylspiperone PET scan at the level of the heads of caudate before (*left*) and after (*right*) the administration of oral haloperidol. Images were taken approximately 45 minutes after injection of the tracer with a NeuroECAT PET scanner (CTI). Both images were scaled to the same intensity maximum and normalized for injected dose. Marked blockade of the uptake of the tracer in the basal ganglia is apparent after Haldol administration.

analysis has both historical and theoretical precedent. Thus, the use of tissue ratios for estimating receptor density and affinity with PET radioligands, as was done with ^{11}C-raclopride by Farde et al. (1986, 1987), may be an acceptable simplification. However, proof of meeting assumptions of quasi-equilibrium is an important factor that needs to be validated. In the case of ^{11}C-raclopride, the initial reports by Farde et al. (1986, 1987) did not include measurement of the input function, labeled metabolites, or analysis of rate constants with a kinetic model. Such studies are currently being carried out with raclopride (L. Farde, personal communication). It is important to note that both of these rather different modeling approaches are variants of analysis of the same three- or four-compartment model. Furthermore, both models require validation of their assumptions, as is described below.

Validation of Assumptions in Quantitative Models

All quantitative models used in PET make a number of assumptions. Such assumptions must be tested for their validity. For example, partition coefficients for oxygen in ^{15}O methods (Frackowiak et al. 1980) and the lump constants for glucose metabolism determined with fluorodeoxyglucose (FDG) (Phelps et al. 1979) have been assumed for many PET studies. Especially in the latter case, these assumptions are not always met, as evidenced by the variation in lump constants in neoplasia or in stroke (Hawkins et al. 1981, 1986).

The amount of available D_2 receptor ligands, haloperidol and NMSP, are important in our multicompartmental model (Wong et al. 1986a) (Figure 6-5). It has been suggested that differences in binding of such ligands to plasma protein may be different in patients and control subjects (Farde et al. 1988). We examined the degree of binding of ^{11}C-NMSP to plasma proteins in normal subjects (95.7 ± 0.36% bound, mean ± SE; $n = 12$) and patients with schizophrenia, bipolar disorder, and other neuropsychiatric illnesses (95.6 ± 0.4% bound; $n = 21$). These recent results indicate that the amount of NMSP that is available for binding to brain D_2 receptors is very similar in patients and normal subjects. It follows that the same should be true for another butyrophenone—haloperidol—which has very similar structure and pharmacology to NMSP. We are currently testing the binding of haloperidol to plasma proteins directly with ^{18}F-haloperidol in patients and control subjects. The fact that patients reported in Wong et al. (1986c) and those studied since (Wong et al. 1989a, 1989b) had normal serum protein and albumin measures and were well nourished as documented by the medical history at the time of the scan (L.E. Tune, personal communication) also argues against

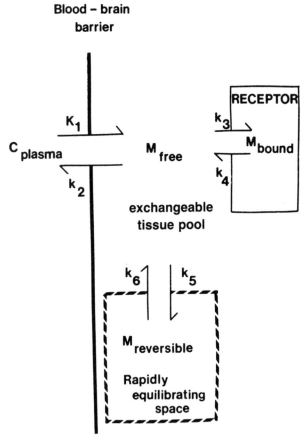

Figure 6-5. Description of the three-compartment model. ^{11}C-Labeled *N*-methylspiperone ([11C]NMSP) first crosses the blood-brain barrier and then binds to the D_2 receptors. ^{c}plasma = concentration of the ligand in arterial plasma; ^{M}bound = quantity of ligand bound to the D_2 receptors; ^{M}free = quantity of drug in the exchangeable pool of the tissue; ^{M}reversible = quantity of drug bound to the other secondary or non-D_2 receptors assumed to be in rapid equilibrium with the free ligand in the brain. K_1 is the clearance from plasma; K_2 is the rate constant for the escape from brain tissue of [11C]NMSP; K_3 and K_4 are rate constants for, respectively, the association and dissociation of the ligand with the D_2 receptors; K_5 and K_6 are rate constants that refer to the lower affinity or secondary rapid reversible binding that is present in the caudate but not in the cerebellum. All PET techniques that quantify neuroreceptors use a similar multicompartmental model to obtain kinetic parameters of binding to neuroreceptors.

differences in protein binding across subject groups. Such studies are crucial, since an accurate estimation of available haloperidol in the brain is necessary in our calculation of D_2 receptor density.

A related assumption involves the partition coefficient for haloperidol between brain and plasma. In studies with ^{3}H-labeled haloperidol (Wong et al. 1986c), partition coefficients for haloperidol were found to be approximately 3 (g brain tissue/ml plasma), which is compatible with previous assumptions. These partition coefficients require special attention because they represent partitioning relative to plasma, whereas total serum haloperidol levels are used in our calculations. Additional experiments are being carried out with ^{18}F-haloperidol to measure the partition coefficient in postmortem brains from control subjects and subjects with various neuropsychiatric disorders.

It is assumed that binding reaches equilibrium in PET studies with reversibly bound radioligands (i.e., equilibrium model). Farde et al. (1986, 1987) measured total binding in D_2 receptors in striatum divided by their estimate of free concentration derived from cerebellar brain values of ^{11}C-raclopride assumed to be at equilibrium. In these studies they did not employ a dynamic model to demonstrate binding equilibrium. We have demonstrated how this can be accomplished (Wong et al. 1986b) with equilibrium binding of ^{11}C-NMSP to cortical 5-HT_2 receptors (quasi-equilibrium is reached because the binding to 5-HT_2, in contrast to D_2 receptors, is reversible). Such analyses require that the complete blood and brain time activity curves (radioactivity plotted against time) are known up until the time that binding ratios are examined. The assumption that equilibrium has been reached, when in fact it has not yet been achieved, may unfavorably alter measurements of receptor density and affinity.

Another important model assumption to consider is the treatment of labeled radioligand metabolites. Knowledge of the concentration of labeled metabolites is necessary to determine the true input function from blood to brain regions containing the neuroreceptors. We previously employed a model correction for metabolites involving the relationship between the volume of distribution of the tracer in cerebellum as it falls relative to total plasma radioactivity (Wong et al. 1986a). Although at that time high-performance liquid chromatography (HPLC) metabolite analysis of the actual blood samples showed good correlation with our model, we have since improved the specificity and sensitivity of HPLC metabolite methods (adapted from Eddington and Young 1988). We have recently examined a large number of patient studies and demonstrated a close relationship between the metabolite and model corrections (Wong et al. 1989a, 1989c). Furthermore, receptor densities calculated with both modeled metabolite corrections and HPLC-measured metabolite corrections, using both blocked (with haloperidol) and unblocked scans, are closely correlated in a number of subjects (Wong et al. 1989a, 1989c). The equilibrium model of Farde et al. (1986) measures brain tissue ratios without blood sampling. They assume a quasi-equilibrium among compartments so that metabolite corrections are unnecessary. However, this is another assumption that needs to be proven by kinetic analysis before simplification to measuring brain ratios can be safely employed. Violation of such model assumptions may contribute to the differences in results obtained from different centers such as the controversy between the Johns Hopkins and Karolinska studies (Andreasen et al. 1988). The assumptions made in any quantitative model must ultimately be validated to ensure the appropriateness of such models.

PET Instrumentation

There are currently numerous different PET scanners available. Newer systems have more rings of detectors and other modifications that can improve the in-plane spatial resolution of structures to less than 5 mm. Such precision is particularly important when very small structures are of interest to the investigator. In the Johns Hopkins and Karolinska studies examining D_2 receptors in schizophrenia, different PET systems are employed, although both systems had similar spatial resolution. Since there is no gross pathology in the striatum in schizophrenia, it is unlikely that equipment differences would be a major factor in interpretation of results. On the other hand, in a neuropsychiatric disorder with marked atrophy, such as Alzheimer's disease, or with striatal degeneration, such as Huntington's disease, PET camera differences may be very relevant. As interest is focused on smaller structures, and as the spatial resolution reaches theoretical limits of PET (a few millimeters), such issues as scatter attenuation correction will become important factors in the determination of abnormalities in disorders as well as variability between research centers.

Anatomical Alignment and Localization

Since neuroreceptor binding determined with PET yields functional images, they must be based on an appropriate anatomical scheme. In both the Johns Hopkins and Karolinska studies, X-ray CT was employed prior to the PET procedure for alignment purposes. At present, both centers have the ability to overlay magnetic resonance imaging or CT scans with PET images with appropriate registration procedures that will improve the placement of regions of interest

(Figure 6-6). In these particular studies of drug-naive schizophrenic patients, regions of interest were determined in different manners: in the Johns Hopkins study, investigators identified peak values in a 2 × 2 pixel area on PET images, whereas a CT overlay was used in the Karolinska study. It is unlikely that the difference in the placement of regions of interest was a significant confounding factor because of the modest resolution of both scanners and the fact that brain structures were relatively easy to examine. Although unlikely to account for the discrepancies between the two studies, these procedures may contribute to the considerable variance in measures of receptor B_{max}. Recent developments in the anatomic localization and placement of regions of interest will diminish this source of variance in future PET neuroreceptor studies.

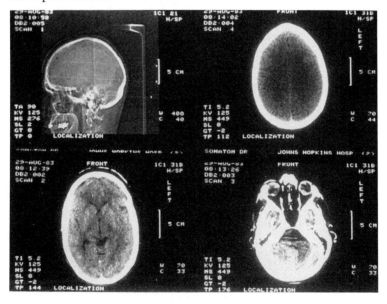

Figure 6-6. Example of anatomical alignment of PET. A topogram obtained in CT scanner illustrates the angle (close to the canthomeatal line using external landmarks) at which transverse images are obtained. The transverse noncontrast CT images illustrate anatomical regions that are imaged with the NeuroECAT PET camera. The three images, 32 mm apart, correspond to the rings of detectors. The *bottom left* image shows maximum volume of heads of caudate that are of interest to dopamine neuroreceptor imaging. The subject wears a rigid thermoplastic mask on which a line is marked to ensure that the PET image is correctly aligned to chosen neuroanatomic regions.

Supportive Evidence From Other Neuropsychiatric Disorders

Although not a direct validation, results from PET studies in other patient groups may give insight into understanding the differing results obtained with PET in cases of schizophrenia. A specific example of this is the study of another neuropsychiatric patient group, bipolar affective disorder. This disorder is of particular interest because of the episodic clinical picture and psychotic symptoms that may occur. Although not the major pathophysiologic hypothesis, there are several lines of evidence that implicate the dopaminergic system in this disorder (Jimerson 1987). In an unpublished work with G.D. Pearlson, we have examined 14 bipolar patients, 7 who were psychotic and 7 who were nonpsychotic at the time of the PET scan. Thus far, psychotic bipolar subjects show elevated D_2 receptor B_{max} values of the magnitude previously published in the drug-naive schizophrenic patients. The nonpsychotic bipolar patients appear to be indistinguishable from the normal control subjects. This apparent separation in mean B_{max} values, if confirmed, suggests that the dopaminergic system may be important in psychosis irrespective of psychiatric diagnosis (Wong et al. 1989b). This makes it unlikely that our findings merely reflect violation of model assumptions. This example should illustrate how findings in another psychiatric disorder can provide corroborative evidence because of potential pathophysiologic similarities with the disorder under investigation.

CLINICAL ISSUES

Future Studies

Our finding of an abnormality in the D_2 receptor in schizophrenia demonstrated by PET illustrates how an important basic science question can be addressed in the living human brain without the limitations of animal models or postmortem human brain tissue. However, it is important to understand potential clinical correlations and implications of any such findings. For instance, a crucial question is whether changes in this neuroreceptor are related to the state of the individual, i.e., psychotic state, or represent a trait abnormality. If elevated D_2 receptor densities as shown with PET are related to the presence of psychosis, it would be important to understand whether elevations are correlated with the degree of psychosis. Furthermore, it is of interest to examine whether D_2 receptor B_{max} falls after symptomatic improvement. Because the mainstay of treatment for schizophrenia is neuroleptics, it may be difficult to tease apart whether any such changes in D_2 receptor B_{max} were due to neuroleptic treatment itself or to the improvement of symptoms. Another potential application would be in the early detection of relapses of psychotic symptoms in these patients. If it could be shown that PET measurement of D_2 receptor B_{max} could detect preclinical changes in B_{max} prior to a relapse of psychotic symptoms, PET might be used to help monitor the chronic treatment of schizophrenic patients to minimize neuroleptic exposure and hence the risk of tardive dyskinesia.

On the other hand, if elevated D_2 receptor densities demonstrable with PET are present throughout the illness, such a test may have potential value as a diagnostic marker and perhaps be of value to predict the illness prior to the first psychotic break. With the renewed interest in a possible genetic marker for schizophrenia (Sherrington et al. 1988), a PET procedure might help to clarify the significance of such a marker. It is also of interest to speculate whether subtypes of schizophrenia could be distinguished by PET D_2 receptor imaging so that treatments could be tailored to the specific subtype of illness. Indeed, Wolkin et al. (1989) presented evidence that suggests PET imaging of dopamine receptors may have value in distinguishing neuroleptic responders and nonresponders.

Such questions are at this point speculative because PET D_2 receptor findings require additional confirmation. Future work in PET will have to address such relevant clinical questions. One area that is under current scrutiny with PET is central D_2 receptor blockade after neuroleptic treatment. Following is a brief outline of three recent studies that have attempted to investigate brain D_2 receptor occupancy with PET and correlate such findings with neuroleptic administration.

Dopamine Receptor Occupancy Studies

It is well established that neuroleptics are effective in the treatment of psychotic symptoms of schizophrenia. Furthermore, it has also been clearly established that typical neuroleptics reliably block central dopamine neuroreceptors in animal studies. What was not possible to demonstrate until PET neuroreceptor imaging was developed was a correlation between dopamine receptor occupancy and neuroleptic treatment in living human brains. Cambon et al. (1987) employed PET with [76]Br-labeled bromospiperone to examine the degree of dopamine receptor occupancy after treatment with various neuroleptics in six psychotic patients. They plotted chlorpromazine equivalent doses and degree of receptor occupancy from two PET scans, on and off neuroleptic treatment, and found a curvilinear relationship between dose and occupancy. They suggested that receptors were almost completely occupied at low doses of neuroleptics and suggested a narrow range of doses that lead to receptor occupancy. Two years later, Wolkin et al. (1989) studied 26 subjects and correlated plasma haloperidol concentration with the degree of receptor blockade using the PET ligand ^{18}F-NMSP. They also found a curvilinear relationship suggesting that maximum blockade was reached with a low blood level of haloperidol. They suggested that their findings were a strong argument in favor of monitoring plasma neuroleptic drug levels. In the same year, Farde et al. (1989) presented evidence from PET scans with ^{11}C-raclopride in eight schizophrenic patients, which suggested that plasma raclopride concentrations, when corrected for degree of protein binding, were linearly related to D2 receptor occupancy in brains over a wide range of concentrations. Findings from these three studies are of great interest but again demonstrate the difficulties in comparing PET studies that employ different techniques and ligands. They suggest that PET may have value in titrating a neuroleptic dose to an individual patient.

DISCUSSION

In this chapter, several important considerations for the design and interpretation of PET neuroreceptor studies were presented (Figure 6-7). Dopamine receptor quantification with PET, especially in schizophrenia, was chosen as an example to illustrate some of these points. It is apparent that different methodologic and clinical issues in various PET centers around the world may result in discrepant findings in the same neuropsychiatric disorder. An example of divergent findings in two PET neuroreceptor studies examining D2 receptors in schizophrenia further illustrates the importance of addressing such issues. The ongoing work of validating model assumptions in both these centers will improve PET neuroreceptor quantification. Patient and control population factors require further study. Differences between experimental approaches could be examined directly by studying the same patient groups with both ligands, as suggested in a recent review (Andreasen et al. 1988). Probably the most compelling explanation for this discrepancy is that NMSP and raclopride may be subject to different pharmacologic factors, such as competition with endogenous dopamine, or that these ligands may bind to different sites. The recent findings by Seeman et al. (1989) and our ongoing studies support such a pharmacologic explanation.

In the brief time that PET neuroreceptor imaging has been applied to the study of neuropsychiatric disorders, numerous intriguing findings have been obtained with various techniques and PET ligands. Although some controversy surrounds findings obtained in a number of disorders, such techniques have increased our understanding of receptors and neurotransmitters in the living brain. It is hoped that continued effort directed at both methodological and clinical issues will help to clarify the role of PET in both research and the clinical practice of psychiatry.

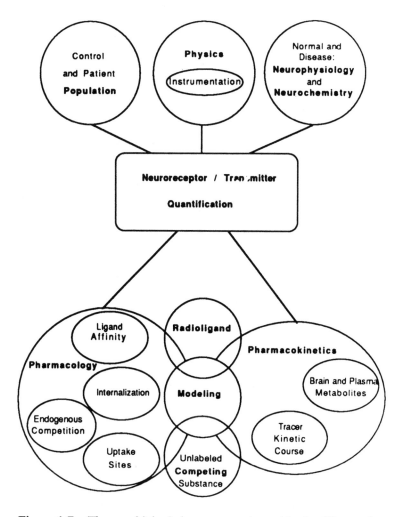

Figure 6-7. These multiple circles represent the multitude of factors that are important for accurate quantification of neuroreceptor binding in the living human brain. Examining the effects of each of these factors can lead to a systematic approach to accurate quantification, and appropriate comparison between different studies can be accomplished.

REFERENCES

American Psychiatric Association: Diagnostic and Statistical Manual of Mental Disorders, 3rd Edition, Revised. Washington, DC, American Psychiatric Association, 1987

Andreasen NC, Carson R, Diksic M, et al: Workshop on schizophrenia, PET, and dopamine D_2 receptors in the human neostriatum. Schizophr Bull 14:471–484, 1988

Arnett CD, Shive CY, Wolf AP, et al: Comparison of three ^{18}F-labeled butyrophenone neuroleptic drugs in the baboon using positron emission tomography. J Neurochem 44:835–844, 1985

Barrio JR, Satyamurthy N, Keen RE, et al: 3-(2^1-[F-18]Fluoroethyl) spiperone: tomographic dopamine characterization in living primates. J Nucl Med 27:879, 1986

Burt DR, Creese I, Snyder SH: Antischizophrenic drugs: chronic treatment elevates dopamine receptor binding in brain. Science 196:326–327, 1977

Cambon H, Baron JC, Broulenger JP, et al: In vivo assay for neuroleptic receptor binding in the striatum. Br J Psychiatry 151:824–830, 1987

Chugani DC, Ackermann RF, Phelps ME: In vivo [3H]spiperone binding: evidence for accumulation in corpus striatum by agonist-mediated receptor internalization. J Cereb Blood Flow Metab 8:291–303, 1988

Comar D, Zaritian E, Verhas M, et al: Brain distribution and kinetics of ^{11}C-chlorpromazine in schizophrenics: positron emission tomography. Psychiatry Res 1:23–29, 1979

Crawley JC, Owens DG, Crow TJ, et al: Dopamine D_2 receptors in schizophrenia studied in vivo (letter). Lancet 2:224–225, 1986

Creese I, Burt DR, Snyder SH: Dopamine receptor binding predicts clinical and pharmacological potencies of antischizophrenic drugs. Science 192:481–483, 1976

Eddington ND, Young D: Sensitive electrochemical high performance liquid chromatography assay for the simultaneous determination of haloperidol and reduced haloperidol. J Pharm Sci 77:541–543, 1988

Farde L, Hall H, Ehrin E, et al: Quantitative analysis of D_2 dopamine receptor binding in the living human brain by PET. Science 231:258–261, 1986

Farde L, Wiesel F-A, Hall H, et al: No D_2 receptor increase in PET study of schizophrenia. Arch Gen Psychiatry 44:671–672, 1987

Farde L, Sedvall G, Wiesel F-A, et al: In reply to: Brain dopamine receptors in schizophrenia: PET problems. Arch Gen Psychiatry 45:599–600, 1988

Farde L, Wiesel FA, Halldin C, et al: In reply to: Dopamine receptor occupancy and plasma haloperidol levels. Arch Gen Psychiatry 46:483–484, 1989

Frackowiak RS, Lenzi G, Jones T, et al: Quantitative measurement of regional cerebral blood flow and oxygen metabolism in man using ^{15}O and positron emission tomography: theory, procedure, and normal values. J Comput Assist Tomogr 4:727–736, 1980

Frost JJ, Mayberg HS, Fisher RS, et al: Mu-opiate receptors measured by positron emission tomography are increased in temporal lobe epilepsy. Ann Neurol 23:231–237, 1988

Hawkins RA, Phelps ME, Huang SC, et al: Effect of ischemia on quantification of local cerebral glucose metabolic rate in man. J Cereb Blood Flow Metab 1:37–51, 1981

Hawkins RA, Phelps ME, Huang SC: Effects of temporal sampling, glucose metabolic rates, and disruptions of the blood-brain barrier on the FDG model with and without a vascular compartment: studies in human brain tumors with PET. J Cereb Blood Flow Metab 6:170–183, 1986

Huang SC, Phelps ME, Hoffman EJ, et al: Noninvasive determination of local cerebral metabolic rate of glucose in man. Am J Physiol 238:E69–E82, 1980

Huang SC, Barrio JR, Phelps ME: Neuroreceptor assay with positron emission tomography: equilibrium versus dynamic approaches. J Cereb Blood Flow Metab 6:515–522, 1986

Jimerson DC: Role of dopamine mechanisms in the affective disorders, in Psychopharmacology: The Third Generation of Progress. Edited by Meltzer HY. New York, Raven, 1987

Kohler C, Hall H, Ogren S-O, et al: Specific in vitro and in vivo binding of ^3H-raclopride. Biochem Pharmacol 34:2251–2259, 1985

Kuhar MJ, Murrin LC, Malouf AT, et al: Dopamine binding in vivo: the feasibility of autoradiographic studies. Life Sci 22:203–210, 1978

Lee T, Seeman P: Binding of ^3H-neuroleptics and ^3H-apomorphine in schizophrenic brains. Nature 274:897–900, 1978

Logan J, Dewery SL, Shive CY, et al: Kinetic analysis of [^{18}F]haloperidol binding in baboon and human brain. J Nucl Med 30:898, 1989

Luchins DJ: Computed tomography in schizophrenia: disparities in the prevalence of abnormalities. Arch Gen Psychiatry 39:859–860, 1982

Lyon RA, Titeler M, Frost JJ, et al: ^{3}H-3-N-Methylspiperone labels D_2 dopamine receptors in basal ganglia and S_2 serotonin receptors in cerebral cortex. J Neurosci 6:2941–2949, 1986

Mackay AVP, Iversen LL, Rossor M, et al: Increased brain dopamine and dopamine receptors in schizophrenia. Arch Gen Psychiatry 39:991–997, 1982

Mayberg HS, Robinson RG, Wong DF, et al: PET assessment of cortical S_2-serotonin receptor binding: lateralized changes following stroke and their relationship to depression. Am J Psychiatry 145:937–943, 1988

Maziere B, Loc'h C, Baron JC, et al: In vivo quantitative imaging of dopamine receptors in human brain using positron tomography and 76Br-bromospiperone. Eur J Pharmacol 114:267–272, 1985

Mintun MJ, Raichle ME, Kilbourn MR, et al: A quantitative model for the in vivo assessment of drug binding sites with positron emission tomography. Ann Neurol 15:217–227, 1984

Owen F, Cross AJ, Crow TJ, et al: Increased dopamine-receptor sensitivity in schizophrenia. Lancet 2:223–225, 1978

Perlmutter JS, Larson KB, Raichle ME, et al: Strategies for in vivo measurement of receptor binding using positron emission tomography. J Cereb Blood Flow Metab 6:154–169, 1986

Perlmutter JS, Kilbourn MR, Raichle ME, et al: MPTP-induced up-regulation of in vivo dopaminergic radioligand-receptor binding in humans. Neurology 37:1575–1579, 1987

Phelps ME, Huang SC, Hoffman EJ, et al: Tomographic measurement of local cerebral glucose metabolic rate in humans with (F-18)2-fluoro-2-deoxy-d-glucose: validation of method. Ann Neurol 6:371–388, 1979

Seeman P, Lee T, Chau-Wong M, et al: Antipsychotic drug doses and neuroleptic/dopamine receptors. Nature 261:717–718, 1976

Seeman P, Bzowej NH, Guan HC, et al: Human brain D_1 and D_2 dopamine receptors in schizophrenic, Alzheimer's, Parkinson's and Huntington's diseases. Neuropsychopharmacology 1:5–15, 1987

Seeman P, Guan HC, Niznik HB: Endogenous dopamine lowers the dopamine D_2 receptor density as measured by [^{3}H]raclopride: implications for positron emission tomography of the human brain. Synapse 3:96–97, 1989

Sherrington R, Brynjolfsson J, Petursson H, et al: Localization of a susceptibility locus for schizophrenia on chromosome 5. Nature 336:164, 1988

Smith M, Wolf AP, Shive CY, et al: Serial [^{18}F]-N-methylspiroperidol

(^{18}F-NMS) PET studies measure changes in antipsychotic drug D_2 receptor occupancy in schizophrenics. J Nucl Med 27:880, 1986

Sokoloff L, Reivich M, Kennedy C, et al: The [^{14}C]deoxyglucose method for the measurement of local cerebral glucose utilization: theory, procedure, and normal values in the conscious and anesthetized albino rat. J Neurochem 28:897–916, 1977

Tewson TJ, Raichle ME, Welch MJ: Preliminary studies with [^{18}F]haloperidol, a radioligand for in vivo studies of the dopamine receptors. Brain Res 192:291–295, 1980

Tune LE, Wong DF, Pearlson GD, et al: D2 dopamine receptors in drug naive schizophrenics: update on 20 subjects. Schizophr Res 2:114, 1989

Wagner HN Jr, Burns HD, Dannals RF, et al: Imaging dopamine receptors in human brain by positron tomography. Science 221:1264–1266, 1983

Welch MJ, Kilbourn MR, Mathias CJ: Comparison in animal models of ^{18}F-spiroperidol and ^{18}F-haloperidol: potential agents for imaging the dopamine receptor. Life Sci 33:1687–1693, 1983

Welch MJ, Mathias CJ, Chi DY, et al: Brain uptake of alkylated and fluoroalkylated derivatives of spiroperidol: ligands for studying dopamine receptors in vivo. J Nucl Med 27:879, 1986

Wolkin A, Brodie JD, Barouche F, et al: Dopamine receptor occupancy and plasma haloperidol levels. Arch Gen Psychiatry 46:482–483, 1989

Wong DF, Wagner HN Jr, Dannals RF, et al: Effects of age on dopamine and serotonin receptors measured by positron tomography in the living human brain. Science 226:1393–1396, 1984

Wong DF, Wagner HN Jr, Pearlson G, et al: Dopamine receptor binding of C-11 3-N-methylspiperone in the caudate in schizophrenia and bipolar disorder: a preliminary report. Psychopharmacol Bull 21:595–598, 1985

Wong DF, Gjedde A, Wagner HN Jr: Quantification of neuroreceptors in living human brain, I: irreversible binding of ligands. J Cereb Blood Flow Metab 6:137–146, 1986a

Wong DF, Gjedde A, Wagner HN Jr, et al: Quantification of neuroreceptors in living human brain, II: inhibition studies of receptor density and affinity. J Cereb Blood Flow Metab 6:147–153, 1986b

Wong DF, Pearlson GD, Tune LE, et al: Update on PET methods for D2 dopamine receptors in schizophrenia and bipolar disorder. Schizophr Res 2:115, 1986c

Wong DF, Wagner HN Jr, Tune LE, et al: Positron emission tomography reveals elevated D2 dopamine receptors in drug naive schizophrenics. Science 234:1558–1563, 1986d

Wong DF, Singer H, Pearlson G, et al: D2 dopamine receptors in Tourette's syndrome and manic depressive illness. J Nucl Med 29:820, 1988

Wong DF, Young D, Young LT, et al: Validation studies of PET D2 dopamine receptor quantification in schizophrenia using [C-11] NMSP. J Nucl Med 30:731, 1989a

Wong DF, Young LT, Pearlson G, et al: D2 dopamine receptor densities measured by PET are elevated in several neuropsychiatric disorders. J Nucl Med 30:731, 1989b